11/07/2005

To Beverly:

With very best regards.

John D Bayn

Medical Errors and Medical Narcissism

John D. Banja, PhD

Clinical Ethicist
Assistant Director of Programs in Health Sciences and Clinical Ethics
Center for Ethics

Associate Professor
Department of Rehabilitation Medicine
Emory University
Atlanta, GA

JONES AND BARTLETT PUBLISHERS
Sudbury, Massachusetts
BOSTON   TORONTO   LONDON   SINGAPORE

World Headquarters

Jones and Bartlett Publishers	Jones and Bartlett Publishers	Jones and Bartlett Publishers
40 Tall Pine Drive	Canada	International
Sudbury, MA 01776	2406 Nikanna Road	Barb House, Barb Mews
978-443-5000	Mississauga, ON L5C 2W6	London W6 7PA
info@jbpub.com	CANADA	UK
www.jbpub.com		

Library of Congress Cataloging-in-Publication Data
Banja, John D.
  Medical errors and medical narcissism / John Banja.
    p. ; cm.
  Includes bibliographical references and index.
  ISBN 0-7637-8361-7 (hardcover)
  1. Medical errors—Psychological aspects. 2. Physicians—Professional ethics. 3. Physicians—Psychology. 4. Narcissism.
  [DNLM: 1. Medical Errors. 2. Narcissism. 3. Physicians—ethics. 4. Professional Autonomy. WB 100 B217m 2004] I. Title.
  R729.8.B36 2004
  610—dc22

                                                                        2004015131

Production Credits
Executive Editor: Jack Bruggeman
Production Manager: Amy Rose
Associate Production Editor: Tracey Chapman
Editorial Assistant: Kylah McNeill
Marketing Manager: Ed McKenna
V.P., Manufacturing and Inventory Control: Therese Bräuer
Composition and Art: Bookwrights
Cover Design: Kristin E. Ohlin
Text Design: Ann Marie Lemoine
Printing and Binding: Malloy, Inc.
Cover Printing: Malloy, Inc.

Printed in the United States of America
08 07 06 05 04   10 9 8 7 6 5 4 3 2 1

Table of Contents

Chapter 7   The Empathic Disclosure of Medical Error   173

JOHN BANJA and GERI AMORI

Chapter 8   Beyond Errors—Beyond Narcissism   193

Appendix 1   Error Rationalization and the Somatically Marking Brain   205

Dedication

This book is dedicated to all healthcare professionals who did the right thing, when doing the right thing was very, very difficult.

This book evolved out of my interest in the psychodynamics of emotionally painful healthcare communications. After teaching and writing on bioethical issues for many years, as well as serving on and working with various hospital ethics committees, I am singularly struck by how often real-life ethical dilemmas emerge as the result of relational breakdowns. While moral philosophers are typically interested in the conceptual subtleties attached to definitions of personhood, justice, and the like, the kinds of ethical dilemmas that routinely occur in hospitals and clinics seem to me essentially different. So very often, when these situations come to an ethics committee for review, the case reflects relational ruptures that are punctuated by a host of painful feelings—especially anger, bewilderment, and intense frustration—that are borne by all the parties. I have come to realize that managing these feelings artfully is a key skill that many healthcare professionals do not possess but that they must master.

This book is concerned with a very familiar psychological experience in healthcare: namely, situations wherein the health professional's feelings of control, adequacy or competence are threatened. These feelings can occur in any number of situations, such as caring for a dying patient, disclosing a patient's unexpected death to his or her family, communicating an anxiety-provoking finding such as a malignant cancer, or disclosing a harm-causing medical error.

Disclosing a harm-causing medical error can be one of the most anguishing conversations a health professional can have, and the anecdotal literature of the twentieth century indicates that it is a conversation that health professionals frequently avoid or conduct poorly. In addition to addressing the fear that the disclosure of an error might lead to a lawsuit, I discuss in the following pages the ways that errors might assault the professional's sense of competency and adequacy, and how that assault might be psychologically intolerable. A psychological construct that I am particularly keen to explore is the idea that a peculiar kind of narcissistic formation can be present among many health professionals, which I call "medical narcissism." The self-protecting nature of narcissistically based defenses explains, I believe, how error disclosure to patients is often compromised by the health professional's need to preserve his or her self-esteem at the cost of honoring the patient's right to the unvarnished truth about what happened.

Chapter One lays the groundwork for the definition of error and describes how errors happen. It ends with a discussion of the occasionally ambiguous nature of error occurrence and the vagaries that sometimes surround whether a poor outcome was or was not caused by error. Those vagaries often provide the health professional with excuses for not disclosing error, even when error is reasonably known to have caused harm.

Chapter Two explores the phenomenon of rationalization, and how its availability is often irresistible to health professionals involved in an error, so that they might feel justified in concealing errors from patients. My friend and colleague, Grena Porto, a past president of the American Society for Healthcare Risk Management, contributed a number of case examples as well as editorial advice to this chapter.

Chapter Three is an exploration of narcissism by way of discussing its healthy manifestations, pathological manifestations, and peculiar appearance among health professionals, especially physicians. Because narcissism is essentially a psychological defense that protects against uncomfortable challenges to a person's sense of self, I show how it is a companion phenomenon to the temptation of rationalization as described in Chapter Two.

Chapter Four offers a case study of error concealment that illustrates a number of themes from the previous chapters, while Chapter Five examines the phenomenon of forgiveness, and why it is an alien construct in healthcare. Because forgiveness requires a humbling of the self, I discuss how narcissistically inclined persons, be they health professionals or patients who are harmed by error, can be "forgiveness challenged."

Chapter Six provides a number of recommendations targeting tort reform, organizational responses to error reporting, and certain kinds of healthcare education that might encourage more ethical conversations about harm-causing error.

Chapter Seven describes the mechanics of the error disclosure conversation itself. Dr. Geri Amori, a past-president of the American Society for Healthcare Risk Management, provided numerous suggestions and editorial recommendations.

Chapter Eight offers some insights on the intersection of truthful disclosure of medical error and overcoming the self-preoccupation and protection that is so typical of the narcissistic character formation.

Much of the material that fills these pages comes from the research, extensive lecturing, and professional conversations I have had with healthcare professionals over the years. Especially important in these efforts is my association with the Georgia Hospital Association Research and Education Foundation (GHAREF) as one of its investigators on a research project that was awarded to it by the Agency for Healthcare Research and Quality (AHRQ) in 2001. I would not have been able to write this book without the opportunity to study errors that became available to me through the support of these organizations. However, the errors contained in this book are mine and mine alone, and none of the opinions expressed in it are necessarily those of the GHAREF nor the AHRQ.

As it is customary in prefaces to give thanks, I must begin with my wife of thirty-three years, Judy, and my sons Mike and Chris— who have very patiently tolerated my narcissism for decades. As always, the staff at the Center for Ethics at Emory, especially its director, Dr. James Fowler, and its associate director, Kathy Kinlaw, have been just as extraordinary in supporting my work as they are extraordinary human beings.

I must also recognize my closest friend, William Morton, MD, JD. For two decades, Bill and I have enjoyed lunch together almost weekly. In addition to being an invaluable source of information and inspiration, his love of learning, immense patience, natural ability as a teacher and raconteur, and his extraordinary love of and zest for life have taught me more than he knows. Thank you, Bill.

I must also thank Jack Bruggeman of Jones and Bartlett Publishers for his enthusiasm, support, and recommendations throughout this project and to Kylah McNeill, Tracey Chapman, and Lydia Horton for their work in editing and producing the book. Also, I must express my gratitude to Dr. Tom Gallagher at the University of Washington for his reading virtually the entire manuscript. His numerous suggestions and his patient efforts to point out my occasional penchant for speculation are very much appreciated.

Last, while this book reflects a compositional effort that occurred over the last two years, much of the manuscript came together during the winter holidays of 2003-2004. For every hour of every day I worked on it, my border collie Dingo was at my side. His alternating expressions of affection, quiet and alert companionship, and blissful sleep (that was frequently punctuated by loud snoring) provided me with a "good enough" environment that I think would have made Donald Winnicott extremely pleased.

John Banja, PhD
Lawrenceville, Georgia

Chapter 1

Error

"The potential for catastrophic outcome is a hallmark of complex systems. It is impossible to eliminate the potential for such catastrophic failure; the potential for such failure is always present by the system's own nature."[1, p. 2]

Richard Cook

Introduction

This first chapter begins with an historical review of medical error communications and explains how a practice of concealing errors took hold as the twentieth century progressed. While the preoccupation of this book is to investigate the phenomenon of medical error concealment despite an acknowledged moral obligation to disclose harm-causing errors, this chapter undertakes the preliminary but important task of exploring various definitions of error that are prominent in the patient safety literature and argues for the adoption of one that appears particularly cogent. The chapter also examines different types of error, their inevitability in human operations, and the systemic nature of catastrophic harm-causing errors. The chapter ends by applying these insights to the phenomenon of error disclosure and shows why such disclosures may be withheld or, when they occur, are often contrived such that they are less than ethical or patient-centered. In short, this first chapter lays the groundwork for comprehending some of the most salient features of error occurrences and offers a glimpse as to how they might affect various ethical and psychological factors associated with harm-causing error disclosure.

To Err Is Human

In June 1998, the prestigious Institute of Medicine (IOM) launched its "Quality of Health Care in America" project. The goal of this 10-year effort aims to secure measurable improvements in Americans' health and on redesigning health delivery for the twenty-first century.[2] The IOM's first report appeared in November 1999. Entitled *To Err Is Human,* this document captured the professional and lay public's attention in a way that few health reports ever had. Occasionally written in a quasi-journalistic style that the authors doubtlessly knew would pique the public's interest, the report began:

> The knowledgeable health reporter for the *Boston Globe,* Betsy Lehman, died from an overdose during chemotherapy. Willie King had the wrong leg amputated. Ben Kolb was eight years old when he died during "minor" surgery due to a drug mix-up.[3, p.1]

The report went on to note, "These horrific cases that make the headlines are just the tip of the ice-berg" and that:

- Over half of all adverse events (i.e., harms or negative outcomes that patients sustained) reported from two large hospital studies resulted from medical errors
- Between 44,000 to 98,000 persons die from medical errors in U.S. hospitals every year, implying that medical errors are at least the eighth leading cause of death in the United States
- Total national costs of medical errors run between $17–$29 billion
- Workplace injuries account for about 6,000 deaths a year, while deaths from medication errors alone account for 7,000
- Hospital costs for medication errors alone run about $2 billion[4]

Once the media got hold of this report, medical errors were at the forefront of the nation's healthcare consciousness. Especially gripping was the media's citing a *New York Times'* characterization of yearly death rates from medical errors as the equivalent of three jumbo jets crashing every two days. "If the airlines killed that many people annually," the *New York Times* reporter observed, "public outrage would close them overnight."[5, p. 26]

In relatively short order, Congress appropriated and delivered $50 million dollars to the Agency for Healthcare Research and Quality to award in the form of research grants whose findings and products would dramatically and rapidly improve patient safety. Congress' appropriation could hardly be faulted. As the IOM report itself acknowledged, errors are responsible for an immense burden of suffering and death; errors should not occur in any case while harm-causing errors especially ought not occur; healthcare lags to the point of embarrassment behind other industries—notably the airlines—that have taken giant steps in reducing harm-causing errors; and the healthcare industry's rapidly growing technological base threatens to cause new errors and harms.

Of central concern to this book, the IOM report notes that the topic of medical errors, "if discussed at all, is discussed only behind closed doors." [p. ix] While that statement might be somewhat exaggerated, it is altogether safe to think that for most of the twentieth century, medical errors were usually concealed from the parties who were harmed, or they were discussed in such a way that no attention was called to the error or to the professional who committed it.

An intentional policy of concealing medical errors appears to have begun in the United States in the late 1920s. Before then, surgeons occasionally published case reports that included mention of their errors. Rosa Lynn Pinkus, who described this period of open acknowledgment of medical error, particularly cites the efforts of Harvey Cushing who inadvertently championed open disclosure of error.[6] Cushing was a leader in establishing neurosurgery as a bona fide medical subspecialty, and he frequently published detailed case reports of his and others' surgical successes and failures. Cushing believed that published clinical accounts that contrasted allowable versus unallowable mistakes or oversights would improve neurological surgery's professional credibility and training standards. He was a firm believer in learning from mistakes, and his patients were sometimes identified in the popular press reports of his work. But all of that changed.

The practice of concealing medical errors evolved from multiple factors. Pinkus writes, ". . . by 1928, the success of the Board of Surgery in its creation of standardized residency programs, the integral use of the scientific method in medical education and the threat of malpractice worked together to prompt a different style of journal reporting."[7, p. 126] As the remainder of this book will discuss, today's malpractice climate can make the healthcare professional's honest disclosure of serious harm-causing errors to the injured party a terrifying, if not foolhardy, affair. Indeed, the last 50 years witnessed physicians receiving a steady stream of advice from supervisors, risk managers, hospital lawyers, and malpractice carriers who stoutly discouraged the truthful disclosure of error. While there is no doubt that serious errors were occasionally disclosed to patients, it seems overwhelmingly true that most harm-causing errors occurring in the twentieth century were concealed. As Beryl Rosenstein, vice president for medical affairs at Johns Hopkins Hospital remarked, "Physicians and nurses are trained from their earliest days in school that health professionals don't make mistakes, and if you do, you don't talk about it (sic)."[8, p.1]

Of course, fear of a malpractice suit is not the only barrier that has a chilling effect on disclosing harm-causing medical errors to patients or their families. As the next chapter will discuss, the realization that an error has seriously harmed a patient is one of the most psychologically painful experiences a health professional can have. Health professionals do not tend to be careless or lackadaisical, and there is little question that the majority of them entered the health professions because of an authentic desire to relieve the pain, misery, and suffering of others. Consequently, when they realize that the individual whose care has been entrusted to them has suffered harm due to error, the psychological impact on the professional can be devastating.[9]

But before a discussion can occur about the nature of error disclosure and the numerous variables that affect it, there needs to be an appreciation of error itself. What is an error, and how should it be defined? A careful definition of error forms a critical backdrop for error disclosure conversations because if a problematic incident turns out not to have been caused by error, then its related communication should proceed differently than if error occurred. But how to define errors? How do they occur? Are they the work of a single person acting ineptly or foolishly, or do harm-causing errors usually require multiple contributors for harm to result? Indeed, a distinction must be made between error and harm, because most mistakes or errors that occur in hospitals have no harmful effect on the patient, while most adverse outcomes or events that occur to hospitalized patients are not the result of error.[10]

This chapter sets the stage for the exploration later in this book of error disclosure. The complex nature of many harm-causing medical errors can create authentic moral ambiguity for the professionals involved who, even in the most unambiguous of circumstances, might blanch at the prospect of communicating error to the patient.

Defining Medical Error: Prominent but Poor Definitions

Prevalent definitions characterize error as a variable of an actor's intention (or lack thereof), either with regard to the actor's behavior or the action's outcome. Lucien Leape's 1994 definition of error is virtually identical with the one adopted by the Joint Commission on Accreditation of Healthcare Organizations (Joint Commission):

> *Leape:* "Error may be defined as an unintended act (either of omission or commission) or one that does not achieve its intended outcome."[11, p. 1851]

> *Joint Commission*: "Error: An unintended act, either of omission or commission, or an act that does not achieve its intended outcome."[12, p. 339]

Consider too how the following definitions are variations on the "intentionality" theme:

> *Dana Farber Cancer Institute:* "Error is an event or act of commission or omission with unintended, potentially negative consequences for the patient."[13]

> *Institute of Medicine* and *The Agency for Healthcare Research and Quality:* "An error is defined as the failure of a planned action to be completed as intended (i.e., error of execution) or the use of a wrong plan to achieve an aim (i.e., error of planning)."[14]

The problem these definitions share is that they disregard the occurrence of factors *that are beyond the actor's reasonable control* but that can nevertheless render his or her action unintentional or that can negatively affect the action's consequence(s).[15] To take a simple example, if Dr. Smith sneezes upon entering a patient's room, is that an error? Suppose this patient is severely paranoid, becomes hysterical, and bolts from the room. Such a "consequence" would certainly count as an unintended outcome of Dr. Smith's unintended sneeze, but would our first inclination be to call the sneeze an "error"? A less fanciful example is this one:

Dr. Jones, who is considered the finest surgeon at Ajax Hospital, is about to repair Mr. Green's abdominal aortic aneurysm. Because Mr. Green has undergone numerous abdominal operations, Dr. Jones realizes that this surgery might be extremely complex because of scarring and anatomical reconfiguration in the surgical site. Although Dr. Jones exercises enormous patience and skill during the operation, he nevertheless lacerates Mr. Green's bowel, which necessitates additional surgery.

Did Jones commit an error? He certainly did not intend to lacerate Green's bowel, nor did he intend for Green to require additional surgery. Although both happened and both fit the error definitions listed previously, most health professionals probably would not ascribe error to Dr. Jones but would call the bowel laceration a "surgical complication" whose possibility Dr. Jones should have discussed in the informed consent conversation with Mr. Green prior to the surgery. Indeed, suppose a group of the best surgeons in the world closely observed Jones during the operation and suppose they unanimously agreed that, given the anatomical complexity of Mr. Green's abdomen, there was virtually nothing Jones could reasonably have done to avert the mishap.

But if, *owing to factors beyond Jones's control*, Dr. Jones could not avoid lacerating the bowel, what sense does it make to say that he "erred"? If analysis shows that it was impossible for Dr. Jones (or any skillful surgeon) to act in a fashion congruent with his intention—or alternatively, if Dr. Jones will invariably do what he does not intend to do (i.e., nick Mr. Green's bowel) because of factors outside his control—what sense does it make to say he erred? The only way Dr. Jones could have avoided error according to the definitions stated above would be not to have done the surgery at all. To blame Dr. Jones for this "error," however, is tantamount to blaming him for not being clairvoyant.

Consequently, it is illogical and unfair to blame Dr. Jones for committing an error because it is unreasonable to hold him to a level of skill that far surpasses what might reasonably be expected of him and his peers. This suggests that while certain unintended acts causing unintended outcomes might be regrettable, some of them ought not count as errors. A good definition of error ought to capture that important point. What follows is an attempt to offer such a definition.

Defining Medical Error: A Better Definition

Err. F(rench) *errer*, L(atin) *errare*, to wander;
Cogn(ate) with goth(ic) *airzeis*, led astray[16, p. 521]
As the etymology of "error" indicates, the root notion of error is "to stray." Now, the previous error definitions would say that the straying consists of a departure from what the actor intends. However, the most beneficent intention performed as well as humanly possible can still go awry. A better explanation is needed for error definition than the one that targets "intention."

In her essay, "Taking Responsibility for Medical Mistakes," Virginia Sharpe offers the following account:

> When we consider medical mistakes and particularly those that cause harm, the blameworthiness of the error depends on how it squares with the obligation of due care. Due care is a legal doctrine that allows that certain individuals may inflict injury while engaged in lawful professional behavior and are liable for damages only if their conduct fails to meet a certain standard of care. In moral terms, if harm results from one's legitimately risky professional conduct, one's blameworthiness depends upon a number of factors related to the reasonable standard of care due or owed. . . Harms associated with recklessness, incompetence, or negligent incapacitation (such as when the practitioner is inebriated) are not genuine "mistakes," since they do not result from error *per se*, but from a disregard for due care itself. When a mistake in reasoning, judgment, or action does involve erring from standards of due care, however, it is a genuine *error* and, as such, is presumed to have occurred within a context of good faith.[17, pp. 184-185]

The strength of defining error according to the standard of care lies in its emphasis on what is "reasonable." Attributing error makes sense only if 1) a standard exists that differentiates erring from non-erring conduct or judgment, and 2) actors can reasonably be expected to know that standard and behave according to it. If no such standard exists, or if a particular situation is such that no one acting in a reasonable fashion could avoid an action that has untoward results, it ought not be said that the person erred.[18] Thus, Dr. Jones did not err in lacerating Mr. Green's bowel because he did all that a reasonably competent surgeon acting in a reasonable manner was required to do. Bad things can happen despite the best intentions carried out in the most competent fashion.

This definition of error, however, is hardly perfect. The weaknesses of a definition of error that rests on the standard of care are that 1) it can be entirely speculative or argumentative as to what the standard of care requires in a given case—indeed, there might not even be such a standard, and 2) even if such a standard exists, there might be no consensus in a given instance as to whether the standard was reasonably followed or violated. Put another way, while the Joint Commission likes the language of "process variation" in studying adverse or sentinel events such as deaths from medication errors, wrong-side or wrong patient surgeries[19, p. 6]—i.e., that a *problematic* variance or departure from the usual and customary occurred in the process of delivering care such that serious harm occurred—experts can argue among themselves over how much a procedure can vary from the norm before it can be authentically labeled a "process variation."

It is important to note, therefore, that the variance, departure, or straying from the standard of care that is presently being offered as a definition of error must be morally problematic, or uncomprehending, or unintended by the actor. Simply calling an error "a failure to accommodate the standard of care" would imply that medicine could not have progressed since Hippocrates without its practitioners making "errors," which seems intuitively wrong. The failure to follow the standard of care, then, must be *unwarranted* and, overwhelmingly, the errors discussed in this book are just so. Intentional "failures" to abide by care standards, which can denote anything from perverse, maleficent behaviors to morally above-board research, constitute a special case of departing from the standard of care that will be discussed in Chapter 6.

The point to be made for now is that it is grossly unfair to hold health professionals to a standard of competence that defines "error" in a way that exceeds ordinary and reasonable levels of performance. Because imputing error can have onerous repercussions, health professionals and especially risk managers must insist on a coherent understanding of error and resist imprecise definitions that could confuse or compromise hospital policy on patient safety and managing adverse outcomes. Consequently, the definition of error that will be used throughout this book is: "An error is an unwarranted failure of action or judgment to accommodate the standard of care."

Performance Failures

A liability of having a neocortex is that humans make errors. In his classic book, *Human Error*, James Reason discusses three types of cognitional failures that sometimes lead to errors: skill-based, rule-based, and knowledge-based.[20] *Skill-based behaviors* rely on perceptual-cognitive-behavioral patterns with which the actor is so familiar that he or she usually performs them in an unconscious or automatic way. These errors often result from "monitoring failures." A good example is when Nurse Jones should have been paying closer attention to what she was doing when she hastily grabbed the wrong patient file or the wrong medication from the pharmacy shelf. These errors are especially common when one's normal routine is disrupted by having to concentrate on doing X where X is non-routine—such as taking one's pet to the veterinarian's office before going to work—so that one neglects to do Y (e.g., remember to take his or her briefcase). Or one might "interchange action schemas," such as catching myself dialing my home phone when I mean to call my office.

Rule-based failures involve either the failure to know the relevant rule, or the misapplication of a good rule, or the application of a bad rule. Thus, a person might carry out an action precisely as planned, but the plan—elegant and competently executed though it was—turns out to be inappropriate to the situation (i.e., a "strong but wrong" plan). Or, a person might follow a very ill-advised rule such as, "When you commit a medical error, never inform the harmed party and always bill them for services connected with the error," only to have that action result in marked patient dissatisfaction or malpractice litigation. Under the revised characterization of error, rule-based failures become errors when a person *ought* to have known what rule was applicable, or *ought* to have known that the rule was inappropriate to the situation or ill-advised.

Knowledge-based errors are the most complex of the three. Here the actor errs because of insufficient information or a misinterpretation of the problem situation. When health providers encounter a novel situation, they can only call upon their experience and hope that they have adequately identified the clinically significant factors of the situation in evolving an action plan. Knowledge-based deficiencies or interpretational errors can obviously lead to serious mistakes. "Errorologists," who are usually cognitive psychologists, have pointed out that health professionals frequently commit knowledge-based mistakes because they are stressed, or they feel immensely pressured by time constraints, or they have a narcissistically based refusal to probe their initial judgments more deeply. Here are three types of knowledge-based mistakes: 1) the availability heuristic, which is using the first information that comes to mind; 2) the confirmation bias, which consists in seeking only evidence that confirms one's plan and dismissing evidence that disconfirms it; and 3) the overconfidence tendency, wherein a person believes in the validity of the chosen course of action without significant justification.[21, p. 1853]

Error Inevitability

When a human being, with his or her imperfect cognitive functioning, is placed in a terrifically complex environment, errors are inevitable. The healthcare environment admits immense technological and sociological complexity. Certain kinds of medical equipment, for example, might not only be difficult to operate, but the monitoring devices in the operating rooms might look similar to, but require a different operating technique from, the ones in the intensive care units. On the other hand, hospital technologies are sometimes not properly maintained, or certain design or operational features are novel, or their assigned practitioners might be inexperienced in using them. Add to all of this the facts that healthcare environments are dynamic and changing; that health professionals rarely have complete information but more often multiple, fragmentary pieces of information delivered with varying degrees of accuracy; that medical decision making is intensely personalized and often relies on judgment calls made under extreme duress; that the actors, whose interdependencies are essential, not only change frequently but exhibit varying levels of competency (thus the old saw among university affiliated hospitals: "Never be admitted to a hospital the first week in July," because that's when the brand new and notoriously inexperienced interns arrive); and that healthcare interventions frequently have multiple and entirely unanticipated consequences to which the professional must nevertheless be prepared to react.[22] Given all of this, Richard Cook dramatically observed:

> The potential for catastrophic outcome is a hallmark of complex systems. It is impossible to eliminate the potential for such catastrophic failure; the potential for such failure is always present by the system's own nature.[23, p. 2]

Cook's emphasis on the "systemic" nature of failure has become central to the contemporary understanding of harm-causing errors and strategies to prevent them, to which the next section will turn.

The Systemic Nature of Medical Error

On February 20, 1995, Tampa surgeon Rolando Sanchez amputated Willie King's left leg.[24] Mr. King's informed consent form and explicit understanding with Dr. Sanchez, however, clearly stipulated the right leg as the one to be removed. The timing of this medical error was as bad as the error itself was astonishing, because state and federal legislatures were in the midst of contemplating various tort reform measures aimed at reducing the number of malpractice suits against physicians as well as reducing their insurance premiums. The fact that a patient could not trust his or her physician to know which leg to amputate not only threw an ugly wrench into those tort reform efforts, but aroused the public's indignation as to how flawed their otherwise much-vaunted healthcare system really was. Needless to say, Dr. Sanchez's career was hardly bolstered by this incident, but as the facts of the wrong-side amputation came out—but were never made available to the public in anywhere near the sensational fashion as the wrong-side amputation itself—Dr. Sanchez looked less and less culpable for the error.

First of all, while Mr. King was certainly not to blame for the error, his case illustrated two common occurrences in wrong-side surgeries: the patient was quite ill, and both his legs (or sides) were in terrible shape.[25] In 1995 Mr. King was a 51-year-old retiree recovering from heart surgery. His medical history was voluminous as he was an insulin-dependent diabetic with a history of severe peripheral vascular disease, peripheral neuropathy, nephropathy, hypertension, coronary artery disease, and severe atherosclerosis. A pre-surgical examination at Tampa University Community Hospital revealed that he had no popliteal pulse in either of his legs. Both legs were cold to the touch and both exhibited gangrenous lesions. Circulation in Mr. King's left leg, that is, the one that was erroneously amputated, might have been more compromised than in his right, because the left leg's arteries appeared almost totally occluded. Mr. King nevertheless wanted his right leg amputated because it was causing him intolerable pain.

Dr. Sanchez, on the other hand, was hardly the buffoon the public took him to be. In 1995, he was 53 years old and at the height of a sterling medical career. He was born in Tampa and attended New York University School of Medicine, where he was chief resident at the Medical Center. While in New York, he taught surgery and was director of the hyperbaric chamber program at Albert Einstein College of Medicine. Martin Hatlie, an attorney who worked with the American Medical Association, characterized Sanchez as a "surgeon's surgeon," while the Florida Agency for Healthcare Administration observed that his reputation was excellent.

Upon examining Mr. King, Sanchez initially recommended bypass surgery, not amputation. Mr. King declined. Later, Sanchez remarked, "I asked the nurse to have the patient sign a consent form for the right leg. It was clear to me, though, that the left leg would need to be amputated in the near future."

The events that followed typified what has become gospel in the contemporary understanding of catastrophic error and are nicely captured in another observation by Richard Cook:

> [T]here is no isolated "cause" of an accident. There are multiple contributors to accidents. Each of these is insufficient in itself to create an accident. Only jointly are these causes sufficient to create an accident. Indeed, it is the linking of these causes together that creates the circumstances required for the accident. Thus, no isolation of the "root cause" of an accident is possible.[26, p. 2]

It is important to note that Cook speaks of "accident" rather than "error." Accident connotes the harm that transpires from error. "Error" on the other hand is an interpretation, label, or characterization of someone's performance that denotes an unwarranted failure to accommodate a particular standard of operation or behavior. People make errors but "systems" can facilitate an error's occurrence, such as keeping medicines that have virtually identical packages side-by-side on the pharmacy shelf. Thus a system can have various faults or "latent failures" that enable errors to occur or that fail to halt an error "trajectory."

The error trajectory of Mr. King's case begins with the initial communication between Dr. Sanchez's office and the operating room scheduler, wherein the operation is officially but incorrectly listed as a left leg amputation. (A reliable explanation of how this "ur-error" occurred has, to this author's knowledge, never appeared.) The multiple contributors to the accident then begin to line up in the form of system failures to intercept this error and halt its catastrophic potential. They include the following:

- The day prior to Mr. King's surgery, a floor nurse notices on her copy of the surgical schedule that Mr. King was scheduled for a left leg operation, which she knows is wrong. She tells a pool nurse about the mistake who then places a corrected copy of the surgical schedule on a clipboard and gives it to another nurse. The change is neither discussed by the nurses as they change shifts nor is the corrected information ever transferred onto the official printed schedule.

- The operating room where Mr. King's surgery is to take place contains a blackboard as well as the official operating schedule. Both incorrectly list Mr. King's surgery as a left leg amputation.

- Shortly before the procedure, a technician arrives to set up the equipment, including the leg holder. Seeing the operation listed both on the blackboard and on the official schedule as a left leg amputation, he sets up the leg holder on the left side of the table.

- Just before his surgery, Mr. King tells the circulating room nurse that his right leg is the correct amputation site. Despite her noting this in the hospital records, she preps the left leg and drapes the rest of Mr. King's body.

- Upon entering the operating room, Dr. Sanchez reviews the incorrect blackboard information and the incorrect surgical schedule while Mr. King is draped and prepped on the wrong sides.
- An Agency for Healthcare Administration hearing officer later noted that the standard of care at that time did not require that a surgeon review the patient's medical records or consent form prior to surgery. Furthermore, it was not a formal part of the standard of care for a surgeon to speak to the patient immediately before surgery so as to confirm the nature of the procedure.

Three-quarters of the way through the operation, the surgical team discovered the error. Mr. King never filed a lawsuit, but the Tampa press reported that the hospital paid $900,000 and that Dr. Sanchez's malpractice insurer paid another $250,000.[27]

The systemic nature of harm-causing error is perhaps the signal finding of errorology research. In a paper that described a "wrong patient" error wherein one patient had the procedure scheduled for another, Mark Chassin and Elise Becher wrote that discrete errors occurred in at least 17 different places.[28] Most notable were communication failures in which, "Physicians failed to communicate with nurses, attendings failed to communicate with residents and fellows, staff from one unit failed to communicate with those from others, and no one listened carefully to the patient."[29, pp. 829–830] The authors noted that these communication failures were remediable so that the probability of future harm occurrence could be reduced. Environmental factors, such as ongoing pressures to reduce the number of staff or perform more invasive procedures on an outpatient basis, are more difficult to resolve, even though they contribute to the frequency of harm-causing errors and certainly contributed to the patient mix-up that Chassin and Becher describe.

The discovery of the systemic nature of harm-causing error is quite startling because it contradicts the more common sense view that a disaster like Willie King's case is the work of one person doing something confoundingly wrong. The prevailing concept that errors would not happen if people were better trained and better motivated turns out to be strikingly false because well-trained, well-motivated people make errors all the time.

Systemic Defenses or the Lack Thereof

Taken together, environmental and latent factors typify complex systems such as healthcare, business, or transportation. These systems tend to be intrinsically hazardous, and therefore *they are heavily defended against failure.* That is, repeated experiences with failure usually lead the system designers and operators to implement layers of defense or redundancy so that an error will be intercepted and its trajectory halted so that it does not result in harm. Thus, the systemic nature of harm-causing error has become the conceptual model for its comprehension, not because of any peculiarity or idiosyncrasy of error itself, but rather because hospitals have implemented layers of defense so that for a harmful error to occur, *it must somehow penetrate these layers*. Notice that at least three opportunities occurred in Willie King's case whereby his wrong leg amputation might have been averted: the failure of the nursing staff to alert the operating room to the scheduling mistake; the failure of the circulating room nurse to note the discrepancy between Mr. King's communication to her and what the operating room team anticipated doing; and Dr. Sanchez's failure to check either Mr. King's chart, informed consent form, or to ask Mr. King to corroborate the surgical plan.

Consequently, in the aftermath of such disasters, the conscientious hospital will explore how the error breached its system's defenses and what additional defenses are required so that a similar accident does not reoccur. Otherwise, a plaintiff's lawyer representing an individual harmed by error likes nothing better than to find that in the months preceding his or her client's injury, multiple patients receiving care at that hospital almost had the same adverse experience, but that someone in the chain of events intercepted the error before it reached the patient. What this says to the plaintiff's counsel is that the hospital appeared to do nothing to repair these system flaws and hence appeared to care little about patient safety.

It is important to reiterate a key finding from the above: No matter how well-designed a system is, errors will happen. They are inevitable given the flaws and imperfections that come with being human. Systems that effectively manage consumer safety therefore will implement ways that make committing an error by system operators more difficult, as well as ways to intercept whatever errors might occur and extinguish their harm-causing potential. When, on the other hand, systems are designed such that a process' constituent tasks are largely disconnected from each other, and whose executions are assigned to individuals working mostly independently from one another, catastrophic harm can indeed result from "single point failures" (i.e., one person failing to do something essential).[30] Surprisingly and tragically, this seems to be precisely what happened in the much publicized 2003 case of Jesica Santillan.

An Absence of System Checks

Eight years to the day after Willie King suffered a wrong leg amputation, 17-year-old Jesica Santillan received a second heart-lung transplant at Duke University Medical Center in Durham, N.C.[31] Thirteen days prior, she received her first transplant but with organs whose A blood type was incompatible with her O type. The error was picked up by a laboratory technician who was performing a routine test. What is especially important to note about this tragedy—Jesica died two days after receiving the second transplant—is that her surgeon, Dr. James Jaggers, appeared to be virtually solely responsible for checking Jesica's blood type against the donor's, despite the fact that numerous professionals coordinated and participated in Jesica's transplant. For example, a United Network Organ Sharing (UNOS) specialist initially fielded a call from a coordinator at the Carolina Donor Services (CDS) who inquired about Jesica's eligibility as an organ recipient. Over the phone, the CDS coordinator incorrectly gave Jesica's blood type as

A, but the UNOS specialist was not required to check it. In addition, the transplant coordinator at Duke was not expected to confirm the blood type of the donor's organs, nor was Dr. Shu Lin, the surgeon who flew from Duke to Children's Hospital in Boston to retrieve the donor's organs. And while the operating room staff at Children's in Boston knew the blood type of their organ donor, they were not required to know Jesica's nor were they required to ask. Indeed, after Lin had taken the organs from the donor, they were placed in a sterile Igloo cooler that was correctly marked with the donor's A blood type.

Much to Duke's credit, the Santillan family was immediately informed of the error. But in what might go down as one of the classic understatements in all of transplant history, Ralph Snyderman, Duke's chief executive was quoted as saying, "We didn't have enough checks."[32, p. 52] In the anguished aftermath of the tragedy, Duke has apparently instituted a dozen separate checks and double-checks of blood type and other medical data, while Duke's transplant surgeons will carry pocket computers that directly link into the hospital's computer system—a technology that Jaggers did not have and that could have prevented the tragedy.

Applications to Disclosing Error

The remainder of this book will explore the health professional's and healthcare organization's reaction to harm-causing error and especially the degree to which error is concealed from or disclosed to the harmed party. Hence, this chapter concludes by enumerating certain lessons that *problematically* bear on error disclosure.

First is whether or not an error actually occurred. The fundamental question, "Was there error?" can be very problematic in certain cases, and its complexity can be compounded because error disclosure can be an anguishing experience that health professionals naturally might be tempted to avoid. Thus the importance of a reliable definition of error and the organization's courage to systematically apply that definition loom large. If there is controversy over applying the terms of any error definition to the factual occurrence itself—for example, the Joint Commission's use of "intention," or this author's reliance on the phrase "standard of care"—a certain amount of interpretational wiggle room will thereby be created for a professional to deny that a harm-causing error occurred. "Rather," he or she might say, "what occurred was a 'complication' or an 'incident,' or an 'unanticipated outcome.'"[33] While a wrong-side surgery, a wrong-patient surgery, or transplanting organs whose blood type is incompatible with the recipient's will not generate controversy about whether or not error occurred, suppose a woman's most recent mammogram clearly shows a cancerous lesion. Her physician inspects her previous year's mammogram and looking at it very, very closely notices a suspicious albeit minute spot on the X-ray. Was it an error to have missed that lesion a year ago, or would virtually any physician, acting in a reasonable and prudent manner, have missed it as well? In this case, the question can ultimately admit no conclusive answer, which can obscure whether or how the putative "miss" should be communicated. However, these kinds of admittedly complex examples, which are hardly uncommon, can easily encourage a *generalized* belief among health professionals that only the most egregious, slam-dunk kinds of mistakes ought to be called errors. The rest might be relegated to an area of questionable "judgment calls," "incidents," or "misadventures," the analysis of which would require too much time to process, not to mention the psychological discomfort that would accompany and thus discourage such an examination. If this assumption is correct, then it suggests that the anxiety generated by this kind of introspection—with its corresponding knee-jerk reflex to discount the incidence of errors—compromises a policy of disclosing harm-causing errors. This will be discussed in much detail in the next chapter.

A second problem concerns the extent to which an obvious error actually caused the adversity a patient experienced. Up to now, this chapter described how an error might not immediately cause harm but is usually coupled with other errors or system failures that ultimately enable harm to occur. Thus, it is well acknowledged that most errors do not cause harm, while most harms that hospitalized patients experience do not result from errors.[34] Whether or not an acknowledged error associated with a patient's bad outcome actually caused that outcome can be immensely speculative. Just as health professionals might feel very uncomfortable about acknowledging an error occurrence, they might be equally inclined to at least question—if not outright deny—that an error caused harm, especially if the patient was already quite ill and his or her adversity could be attributed to any number of factors. (In fact, there was some speculation that the wrong blood might not have been the primary cause of Jesica Santillan's death.) As with the problem of defining error, the causational role of an error might be obscure and call for sensitive and thoughtful communication strategies that will be presented for consideration in later chapters.

Nevertheless, if it is uncertain whether the error contributes to the patient's adverse outcome, it is easy to see how some health professionals might use that uncertainty to excuse their unwillingness to own the error and discuss it openly. Indeed it is quite probable that many health professionals admit to a harm-causing error only in instances where it is absolutely clear that no other factor could have possibly caused the harm. A case example of this phenomenon is presented in Chapter 4.

A third problem involves assigning responsibility. If, as errorologists argue, ". . .overt catastrophic failure occurs when small, apparently innocuous failures join to create opportunity for a systemic failure," then it will not be unusual for an error trajectory to have numerous system operators, such as in the case of Jesica Santillan or Willie King. This creates at least two possibilities among the system operators' reactions to a harm-causing error: The system operators can rapidly quit the scene and stoutly deny any significant responsibility as in, "No snowflake takes responsibility for the avalanche," or they can blame one another. The possibility of blame shifting sometimes creates a serious institutional challenge in trying to construct a coherent, accurate account of what actually happened as well as in keeping staff professionally and emotionally together. Needless to say, if these efforts occur against a backdrop of litigation with multiple staff named in the lawsuit, the challenge can take on Herculean proportions.

If, therefore, these three problematic features of error—its definition, the probability and severity of its harm causation, and allocating responsibility—are exacerbated by the anguish, horror, fear, and guilt that the involved professionals may be feeling, it is quite understandable why the history of medical error has largely been a history of concealment.

For the future of error disclosure to proceed in an honest and ethical way, organizations will have to maintain mechanisms that rigorously investigate putative error occurrences, objectively determine whether an error occurred and caused harm and, in affirmative instances, implement an organizationwide policy that courageously recognizes the harmed party's right to know about harm-causing errors. If many errors occur against a backdrop of ambiguity as to whether an action really was an error, whether the action really caused harm, or who was to blame for action, then it becomes understandable how only the most unambiguous errors might be organizationally acknowledged.

Last, when one factors in the very common psychological tendency of everyone to protect his or her self-esteem along with a natural resistance to self-incrimination in front of patients, the temptation to conceal probable and even categorical errors becomes all the more powerful. Furthermore, and as will be shown in the next chapter, healthcare interventions and outcomes frequently offer themselves up to multiple meanings or interpretations depending on each individual's comprehension of the event. The health professional who is convinced that he or she has much to lose in disclosing a medical error might ascribe moral meanings to an obvious harm-causing error in such a way that he or she can be excused from having to disclose it. The surgical death from error might become a "blessing in disguise," while the professional might convince him- or herself that the blameworthy party in the error scenario was really the patient, whose poor health status augmented the error's harmfulness.

The point of all this is to appreciate how the psychological and epistemological trappings of medical errors can compromise a health professional's customary willingness to discuss information with patients. There is usually considerable room for interpretation in error scenarios—*interpretations that can invite distortion and confabulation* and that allow health professionals to convince themselves that what "really" happened was different from what "appeared" to happen, or that what happened was not as bad as it might seem. Indeed, the remainder of this book is largely an extended reflection on how that interpretational room should be morally managed.

Conclusion

The topic of medical error is like a spider's web: pull one strand and the whole moves. Attempts to define error lead to considerations of medical epistemology and the inevitability of human imperfection. Imperfections in knowledge and performance, especially in high stakes professions such as healthcare, demand the implementation of fail-safe operations that diminish the incidence of errors or the gravity of the harm they cause. When these systemic defenses are absent, such as in Jesica Santillan's case, the occurrence of harm-causing errors is virtually guaranteed. But implementing multiple layers of defense, each with its own system operator(s), results in multiple parties being implicated, if not deemed responsible, when errors penetrate the system's defenses and cause harm. The diffusion of responsibility that naturally follows from adding redundancies to the system can then create significant confusion and dissension as individuals become defensive about their role in and culpability for error. Last, a natural aversion to acknowledgment and disclosure of medical error complicates the psychological formations of health professionals themselves who, after all, can rely only on those formations to get them through the anguish of managing harm-causing error. When there is any question at all about whether an error occurred, the natural self-protective tendency to insulate oneself from organizational or legal penalties can easily incline the individual to use a host of uncertainty factors to justify error concealment.

This opening chapter underlines the nature of complex systems that demand thoughtful understanding of their constituent features so as to manage the moral and operational dimensions of systemic failures. Organizational intelligence must be in place to support health professionals who are involved in committing an error. The ease of committing an error is equally matched by the ease of bungling its aftermath, in terms of damage control, related legalities, and public communications. This book leaves the technological dimensions of error management—that is, superior surveillance, monitoring, equipment maintenance, equipment design, staff training, and so on—to other commentators. The chapters that follow concentrate on the ethics surrounding errors, by exploring how rights, obligations, and normative beliefs play out in a highly complex and stressful environment that sits precariously on the cusp of healing and harming. Add to all this the immense power and social prestige that health professionals command and the way harm-causing error assaults that power and prestige, and it becomes easy to understand how harm-causing medical error can conspicuously expose the darker facets of an entire culture.

References

1. Cook, Richard. *How complex systems fail: being a short treatise on the nature of failure; how failure is evaluated; how failure is attributed to proximate cause; and the resulting new understanding of patient safety.* University of Chicago: Chicago, IL, 1998. Available from ri-cook@uchicago.edu.

2. Kohn, Linda T.; Corrigan, Janet M.; and Donaldson, Molla S. *To Err Is Human: Building a Safer Health System.* Washington, DC: National Academy Press, 2000.

3. Kohn, Corrigan, and Donaldson, 2000.

4. Kohn, Corrigan, and Donaldson, 2000.

5. De Ville, Kenneth, and Elliott, Carl. "To err is human: American culture, history, and medical error," in *Margin of Error: The Ethics of Mistakes in the Practice of Medicine,* Susan B. Rubin and Laurie Zoloth, eds., Hagerstown, MD,: University Publishing Group, 2000, pp. 25–35.

6. Pinkus, Rosa Lynn. "Mistakes as a social construct: An historical approach." *Kennedy Institute of Ethics Journal.* 11(2):117–133, 2001.

7. Pinkus, 2001.

8. Miller, Mary Ellen. "Blame it on the system." *DOME.* 53(4):1–2, 2002.

9. Wu, Albert W.; Folkman, Susan; McPhee, Stephen J.; and Lo, Bernard. "How house officers cope with their mistakes." *Western Journal of Medicine.* 159(5):565–569, 1993; Christensen, John F.; Levinson, Wendy; and Dunn, Patrick M. "The heart of darkness: The impact of perceived mistakes on physicians." *Journal of General Internal Medicine.* 7(July/August):424–431, 1992.

10. Leape, Lucien L. "Error in medicine." *JAMA.* 272(23):1851–1857, 1994.

11. Leape, 1994.

12. Joint Commission. *2002 Hospital Accreditation Standards.* Oakbrook Terrace, IL: Joint Commission on Accreditation of Healthcare Organizations, 2002.

13. Dana Farber Cancer Institute. "Policy for disclosing medical errors to patients and families." Available from Dana Farber Cancer Institute, 44 Binney Street, Boston, MA, 02115.

14. Kohn, Corrigan, and Donaldson, 2000. The February 2, 2001, request for applications from the Agency for Healthcare Research and Quality used language identical to the Institute of Medicine's: "Medical error—the failure of a planned action to be completed as intended or the use of a wrong action to achieve an aim." Available at http://www.AHRQ.gov or from AHRQ's Publications Clearinghouse, P.O. Box 8547, Silver Spring, MD 20907–8547.

15. The errorologist James Reason recognized this in his definition of error: "Error will be taken as a generic term to encompass all those occasions in which a planned sequence of mental or physical activities fails to achieve its intended outcome, and when these failures cannot be attributed to the intervention of some chance agency." The "intervention of some chance agency" implies the point the author wants to make about the insinuation of variables that are beyond the actor's control. See Reason, J. *Human Error.* Cambridge, UK: Cambridge University Press, 1990, p. 9.

16. Weekley, Ernest. *An Etymological Dictionary of Modern English.* Volume One. New York: Dover Publications, Inc., 1967.

17. Sharpe, Virginia A. "Taking responsibility for medical mistakes," in Rubin and Zoloth, 2000, pp. 183–192. Assuming that the standard of care is the one determined by reasonable and prudent health professionals, Albert Wu and his colleagues also offer a definition centering on the standard of care: "We define a medical mistake as a commission or an omission with potentially negative consequences for the patient that would have been judged wrong by skilled and knowledgeable peers at the time it occurred, independent of whether there were any negative consequences." Wu, Albert W.; Cavanaugh, T. A.; McPhee, Stephen J.; Lo, Bernard.; and Micco, G. P. "To tell the truth: Ethical and

practical issues in disclosing medical mistakes to patients." *Journal of General Internal Medicine.* 12:770–775, 1997.

18. Lane, Robert E. "Moral blame and causal explanation." *Journal of Applied Philosophy.* 17(1):45–58, 2000.

19. Joint Commission. *Root Cause Analysis in Health Care: Tools and Techniques.* Oakbrook Terrace, IL: Joint Commission on Accreditation of Healthcare Organizations, 2000.

20. Reason, 1990.

21. Leape, 1994.

22. Cook, Richard, and Woods, David. "Operating at the sharp end: The complexity of human error." *Human Errors in Medicine,* Marilyn Sue Bogner, ed. Hillsdale, NJ: Lawrence Erlbaum Associates, 1994, pp. 255–310.

23. Cook, 1998.

24. All of the material regarding the Willie King wrong leg amputation case is taken from Crane, Mark. "When a medical mistake becomes a media event." *Medical Economics.* 74(11):158–162, 165–168, 170–171, 1997.

25. Crane, 1997.

26. Cook, 1998.

27. Crane, 1997.

28. Chassin, Mark R., and Becher, Elise C. "The wrong patient." *Annals of Internal Medicine.* 136(11):826–833, 2002.

29. Chassin and Becher, 2002.

30. All of the material regarding the Jesica Santillan blood type error is taken from Comarow, Avery. "Jesica's story." *U.S. News & World Report,* July 28/August 4: 51–54, 56, 58, 60, 62, 66, 68, 70, 72, 2003.

32. Comarow, 2003.

33. Finkelstein, Daniel; Wu, Albert W.; Holtzman, Neil A.; and Smith, Melanie K. "When a physician harms a patient by a medical error: Ethical, legal, and risk-management considerations." *The Journal of Clinical Ethics.* 8(4):330–335, 1997.

34. Leape, 1994.

Chapter 2

Rationalization

John Banja
Grena Porto

"We can deny that we committed these wrongs at all. We can insist on a re-description of the wrongs, using a different set of concepts and representing the events as things "happened," as phenomena with no contribution from our human agency. . . The scope for self-protective intellectualizing is tremendous."[1, p. 147]

Trudy Govier

Introduction

This chapter begins with a description of the health professional's psychosomatic response to error, and follows with a discussion of the moral arguments that recommend error disclosure to the harmed party. We will then examine what professionals have reportedly done to manage their reaction to error, despite their moral obligations as defined by ethicists and professional organizations. Because it is known that medical errors are often concealed—or not entirely disclosed—to patients, a central preoccupation of this chapter is to explain the phenomenon of error concealment or semi-concealment and speculate on how a health professional might try to justify a less-than-truthful disclosure of error to the harmed party. Two complementary models bearing on psychological findings will be offered to explain the process and structure of error rationalization with a third, considerably more speculative, neurophysiological model offered as Appendix 1.

The Emotional Response to Medical Error

In her interviews with nurses who committed medication errors, Zane Robinson Wolf summarized her findings by saying:

Some of the nurses interviewed reacted physically and emotionally when they realized they had made a medical error. Some nurses cried; some sobbed hysterically. Their immediate fear of harming or killing the patient propelled some into a stress reaction with physical symptoms: they described the experience as earth shattering and leaving them feeling upset and nervous, or hot all over ... These anxious and panicked nurses feared the possible personal repercussions of the mistake: of losing their jobs, of lawsuits, of having co-workers who would not trust them, and of facing their own incompetence.[2, p. 40]

Similarly, John Christensen and his colleagues interviewed physicians and asked them to recall some of their medical errors and what they remembered their reactions to be. Here are three descriptions:

- I was really shaken. My whole feelings of self-worth and abilities were basically profoundly shaken.
- My great fear was that I had missed something, and then there was a sense of panic.
- It was hard to concentrate on anything else I was doing because I was so worried about what was happening, so I guess that would be anxiety. I just felt terrible; I felt guilty, sad, had trouble sleeping, wondering what was going on.[3, p. 426]

While these quotes might evoke sympathy for the health professionals, it is also comforting to hear their visceral reactions to their mistakes. After all, the physician or nurse who nonchalantly dismisses a serious error or who is utterly numb to its occurrence and consequences is hardly the person patients would want to treat them.

What is very interesting and an important aspect in studying reactions to medical error is the way health professionals prioritize their concerns upon realizing that an error happened. Here are two examples that typify these reactions:

- What if she's really sick and I've really missed it and she's bought the farm because I've waited a year to find this? That's the first thing. And then there's that thought of "What if other people find out? What if the patient finds out?" And then after that sort of a thing like, "What if I got sued for this?"[4, p. 426]
- If something goes wrong with a patient ... the things that come to the doctor's mind are "Was it something I prescribed? Was it an instruction I failed to give? Did I do something wrong?" You get that sinking feeling probably on a daily basis almost.[5, p. 1003]

These quotations suggest a temporally tight juxtaposition of immense anxiety and concern for the patient's welfare, followed closely or even simultaneously by the provider's intense anxiety about his or her own welfare. The lock-step nature of these dual anxieties is key to the discussion that follows.

What Professionals Are Advised About Communicating Error

Regulatory and Insurance Recommendations

Short of requiring that health professionals not lie to patients who have been harmed by error, no national consensus presently exists on how truthfully or comprehensively health professionals should communicate instances of harm-causing error to the harmed parties. A *de minimus* disclosure requirement, for example, is standard RI.1.2.2 of the Joint Commission on the Accreditation of Healthcare Organizations (Joint Commission), which states that "Patients and, when appropriate, their families are informed about the outcomes of care, including unanticipated outcomes." Instances of a patient's experience of serious harm from error obviously fall under this standard, which is further elaborated by the Joint Commission to mean:

> The responsible licensed independent practitioner or his or her designee clearly explains the outcome of any treatment or procedures to the patient and, when appropriate, the family, whenever those outcomes differ significantly from the anticipated outcomes.[6]

The vagaries of this standard involve the meaning of "clearly explains." Depending on how the practitioner interprets the word "explains," a communicator might simply choose to clarify the nature of the outcome: "Mrs. Jones, what happened was that your blood pressure unexpectedly dropped, which explains why you became unconscious and had to be transferred to the intensive care unit." On the other hand, "explains" might be taken to mean that the professional ought to provide a *causal* account of what happened, such as: "Mrs. Jones, what happened was that you had a bad reaction to the medicine we gave you, which resulted in your blood pressure dropping." Notice, however that the Joint Commission standard does not require that the professional utter the words "error" or "mistake" in the communication. Thus it is one thing—and some might argue, not a lie—to tell Mrs. Jones that she had a bad reaction to the medicine she took; it is quite another thing to say, "Mrs. Jones, what happened was that your blood pressure dropped unexpectedly this morning because you were given too much medicine by mistake." The signal difference between these disclosures, of course, is that the latter frankly acknowledges a mistake as a causal element in the patient's adverse event. The Joint Commission however, does not require that health professionals utter the words "error" or "mistake" in communicating an unanticipated outcome caused by error.[7]

Compounding this vagary over how much to disclose are the recommendations from the health professional's insurance carrier, whose historical position when instances of wrongdoing or negligence are suspected has been to advise the insured not to admit "liability" or responsibility for any wrongdoing. Thus, a newsletter from a prominent malpractice carrier that was mailed to thousands of physicians in 2002 suggested that in discussing instances of unanticipated outcomes with patients or their families, the professional should offer a simple explanation of the known facts, explain the known cause of the problem as accurately as possible without speculation, but "not use words which might imply negligence (e.g., error, wrong, mistake, accident)." [8, p. 4]

Driving home this recommendation in a more chilling manner is the fact that many malpractice insurance policies contain a clause that states: "The insured shall not, except at his own cost, make any payment, admit any liability, settle any claims, assume any obligations, or incur any expense without the written consent of the company."[9, p. 416] This "non-cooperation" clause has a prohibitive effect on many error disclosures because the frank admission of a harm-causing error is indeed an admission of liability. The comprehensively honest disclosure of harm-causing error arguably risks the possibility of the insurer's refusal to cover whatever associated costs, principally from a malpractice suit, might occur to the insured. On this account, the health professional's truthful disclosure amounts to a contractual violation of the insurance policy. So great is this fear of the insurer's abandonment of the insured for admitting liability that six states as of this writing have passed legislation that disallows plaintiffs from admitting into evidence at trial the physician's saying, "I'm sorry," as proof of his or her negligence.[10] Indeed, in April 2003, Colorado went even further by disallowing the professional's admission of fault (e.g., "This error caused this adverse outcome") as evidence of negligence.[11]

Ethical Obligations

Now turn attention to a more ethically conscientious body of recommendation on error disclosure, as occurs in section 8.12 of the Council on Ethical and Judicial Affairs *Code of Medical Ethics: Current Opinions,* which states:

> It is a fundamental ethical requirement that a physician should at all times deal honestly and openly with patients. Patients have a right to know their past and present medical status and to be free of any mistaken beliefs concerning their conditions. Situations occasionally occur in which a patient suffers significant medical complications that may have resulted from the physician's mistake or judgment. In these situations, the physician is ethically required to inform the patient of all the facts necessary to ensure understanding of what has occurred. Only through full disclosure is a patient able to make informed decisions regarding future medical care.
>
> Ethical responsibility includes informing patients of changes in their diagnoses resulting from retrospective review of test results or any other information. This obligation holds even though the patient's medical treatment or therapeutic options may not be altered by the new information.
>
> Concern regarding legal liability that might result following truthful disclosure should not affect the physician's honesty with a patient.[12, pp. 217–218]

Like the Joint Commission standard, this requirement does not oblige the professional to say "error" or "mistake," although it is hard to see how the patient can be provided with "all the facts necessary to ensure understanding of what has occurred" and yet have an admission of error withheld. A common sense reading of the section's emphasis on honesty and openness reasonably implies that the discloser admits error or uses words that unambiguously admit mistake, when errors or mistakes are known to have occurred.

Indeed, if the moral objective of disclosure is to respect the patient's right "to make informed decisions regarding future medical care," then it seems correct to say that a *de minimus* compliance with the Joint Commission standard—that is, a disclosure that omits calling attention to an error—would compromise the patient's right to know what happened. An error disclosure policy based on a *patient-centered* perspective, which grounds the ethical basis of disclosure, would be exquisitely truthful, prompt, and comprehensive, assuming this is what the patient wants. And indeed, most patients do. All of the surveys of what individuals want to know in the event of error uniformly find that patients want a truthful account of what happened, and the more serious the outcome, the more elaborate an explanation they want.[13] Furthermore, in addition to apology, individuals harmed by error want assurance that the hospital or professional has made an operational correction or system improvement so that the error does not re-occur.[14]

Disclosure as a Contractual Obligation

In another publication, I argued that the most persuasive explanation for endorsing a patient-centered model of disclosure is to think of the health professional-patient relationship as a contract.[15] While doing so might seem to dismiss the beneficently based understanding of healthcare throughout the ages, the contemporary nature of managed care has unfortunately injected a certain anonymity into the professional-patient relationship—patients often do not know their physicians, who just as often do not know their patients—while the very services that patients claim as a right are largely dictated by the health insurance policy, that is, a contract that the patient has purchased.

The essence of a contractual relationship resides in its usually reciprocal promissory agreements emphasizing obligation.[16] Formal contracts insist on promise-keeping by setting terms that recognize and usually penalize nonperformance. And while this might sound like a reiteration of the trust and fidelity dimensions of the professional-patient relationship articulated in the American Medical Association (AMA) Code of Ethics, it is considerably more. When Jack enters into a contractual relationship with Jill, Jack is not only able to trust and have faith that Jill will perform, Jack has a right to anticipate Jill's competent performance as implicit in Jack's ability to penalize Jill per the contract's terms for nonperformance. The "duty of future performance" dimension of contracts gives legal force to the contractors' ethical commitments resting on trust. Indeed, one of the reasons why legal contracts exist is because contractors might be uncomfortable "only" trusting one another; rather, they want an agreement that binds them with legally enforceable obligations.[17]

Consider that by virtue of their licensure and certification, health providers present themselves to the public as reasonably skilled and competent. Indeed, some commentators suggest that this public "holding forth" of competence is the essence of licensure, which functions as a public notice that even though a patient might have to assume certain risks of harm in agreeing to a course of treatment provided by the professional, *one risk the patient will not have to bear is the risk of harm from substandard care.*[18] Put otherwise, it seems abundantly fair to say that licensed health professionals uniformly agree that the least their patients should expect from them is care whose adequacy meets the professional standard. But if the definition of error as given in the first chapter is correct—namely, that error consists in an act or judgment that, without sufficient warrant, fails to meet the professional standard—then the occurrence of an unambiguous and serious harm-causing error implies that the care was indeed substandard. The professional therefore who does not disclose the error to the harmed party—and notice that the error itself is already a violation of the contract—embarks on a continuing misrepresentation of competence to the very person who had a contractual right to expect that a serious, unambiguous error would not occur. If the error remains concealed, the contractual relationship between patient and professional proceeds under a gross falsehood. Not only has the patient experienced precisely what he or she contractually understood would not occur—namely, harm from substandard care— but he or she is subsequently led down a path of misrepresentation about the quality of care rendered because of the professional's failure to deal honestly and openly about the error. Deprived of the knowledge as to what caused his or her adversity, the patient might believe that he or she is personally responsible for the harm or that it was an "act of God." Furthermore, because of the informational omission, the patient cannot make truly informed decisions about the remainder of his or her care, such as whether he or she wishes to be moved to a different hospital, or make a change of health professionals.

Now, if this argument stopped there, it would appear to rest precisely on a violation of the trust and fidelity dimensions of professional relationships that ethicists and the AMA code underscores. But a second, more contractually rooted dimension follows. Although healthcare providers traditionally enjoy "no fault" agreements with insurers for payment of whatever costs are associated with medical errors,[19] it would be naïve, indeed ludicrous, to assume that the patient harmed by error would similarly excuse error operators and readily pay his or her share of the healthcare bill (e.g., a deductible, co-pay, or the costs of any treatment being denied by his or her insurer) that would additionally accumulate from the error. While health professionals might gloss over the moral significance of patients paying a share of the professional's reimbursement because professionals usually submit their bills directly to the patient's insurer, they cannot deny that most patients today pay a substantial part of their healthcare costs out-of-pocket. But the most fundamental ethical intuition would indict as *fraudulent* the professional who fails to inform a patient of a harm-causing error but then proceeds to accept a fee from the patient for charges related to that error. Under a contractual approach, a patient would demand that the professional remedy his or her performance failure by acknowledging it and offering to make restitution—an offer that a number of hospitals have incorporated into their error disclosure policies by inform-ing parties harmed by error that the costs associated with the error will be removed from their bills.[20]

But even if the individuals associated with the error quietly withdraw those charges from the patient's bill, their ongoing concealment of the error exposes them to a third aspect of this argument: namely, that the patient has a right to recover what-ever financial losses attach to pain, suffering, physical impairment, cognitive dys-function, or death resulting from error.[21] Of course, these monies are precisely what plaintiffs seek to recover when they sue health providers in tort. But defendants who proceed with litigation usually allege that no malpractice was committed and thus no damages should be awarded. The point is that when it is abundantly clear that not only did harmful error occur, but that it caused the harmed party additional expenses from treatments required because of the error, error concealment effectively imposes these additional costs onto the harmed party—and this qualifies as yet another fraudulent breach of contract.

Professionals who oppose error disclosure sometimes justify concealment with an argument to the effect that, "Telling patients or their families about the error would only increase their suffering. They're miserable and unhappy about the poor treatment out-come, so why exacerbate their misery by telling them about the error?" The best reply to this is to ask the health provider to put him- or herself in the role of the harmed patient: "If you were the patient who was seriously harmed by a medical error, would you want to know? If you died as a result of medical error, would you want your family to know? If you were a family member whose loved one was harmed by error, would you want to know?" Perhaps the reason why one study found 98 percent of those surveyed responded affirmatively to these questions is because they are outraged over bearing a cost they have not contractually agreed to pay.[22] Moreover, concealing a fatal harm-caus-ing error might deny persons their right to recover an accidental death benefit they might carry in their insurance.[23, p. 44]

Consequently, error disclosure to the harmed party is ethically mandatory because it respects both the fiduciary as well as contractual nature of the professional-patient rela-tionship. Patients should be able to trust their physicians to inform them about anything that materially affects their care and welfare; patients have the right to make decisions about their medical care, which they cannot exercise with incomplete or deceptive infor-mation; and any financial costs that accrue from error ought not be borne by the harmed party, which in certain instances will require disclosure by the provider. In all of this and as noted by the AMA, ethical obligations that bear on the welfare of the client must trump legal concerns that bear on the welfare of the professional. Because ethical behav-ior is essentially other-regarding and other-directed, an institution's error disclosure policy that leaves a substantial proportion of its listeners in the dark as to whether the harm they experienced did or did not result from error is clearly unethical. It posits the welfare of the health professional over the welfare of the patient, as the only reason for concealment is to protect the professional's interest.[24]

How Do Professionals Actually Communicate Error?

In the event of a harm-causing error, health professionals can either lie or refuse to discuss the error; or they can factually explain what happened but in a way that does not call attention to the error or to themselves as wrongdoers; or they can frankly admit the error and explain its causal role in the patient's untoward outcome.

In a 1997 paper published in the *Journal of Clinical Ethics*, Daniel Finkelstein and his colleagues claimed that physicians most commonly responded to harm-causing error by withholding information associated with the error (or offering incomplete information), by lying, or by avoiding discussion of the outcome.[25] In the same issue of that journal, however, Matthew Sweet and James Bernat reported their survey of physician's self-reported error disclosure practices.[26] They found that, "[P]hysicians generally are willing to admit an error to the patients they are treating. However, as the severity of the injury increased, their willingness to admit an error decreased correspondingly."[27, p. 345] The latter paper stated, "96 percent of the house officers responded that they would tell a patient of an error when the error led to short-term pain, and 78 percent indicated that they would report the error when it [led] to the patient's death."[28, p. 345] Sweet and Bernat cautioned, however, that their study asked physicians what they thought they would do in the instance of harm-causing error, not what they actually did in error scenarios in which they were involved. Thus, it is not known with any precision how errors were communicated, such as whether the words "error" or "mistake" were actually used.

It is pertinent that these studies came out in 1997, given the publication in 1999 of the Institute of Medicine's study *To Err Is Human,* which called international attention to the incidence and frequency of medical errors and placed the phenomenon of error in the health policy spotlight.[29] This document triggered millions of federal research dollars for patient safety research and doubtlessly was a stimulus for the July 1, 2001, Joint Commission regulations on communicating unanticipated outcomes. Given the way today's sensibilities have been shaped by these developments, along with the impact of regulatory standards and the media's heightened interest in reporting catastrophic errors, deceptive communication practices are publicly repudiated. Yet, it is well known that many medical errors or preventable harms remain undisclosed. A 2002 study of disclosure practices reported from over 200 hospitals stated:

> More than half of respondents reported that they would always disclose a death or serious injury, but when presented with actual clinical scenarios, respondents were much less likely to disclose preventable harms than to disclose non-preventable harms of comparable severity. Reluctance to disclose preventable harms was twice as likely to occur at hospitals having major concerns about the malpractice implications of disclosure.[30, p. 73]

What is especially disturbing about this study was the very small number of disclosures that were actually reported in contrast to empirically based estimates of the occurrences of preventable harm—or as the study defined it, ". . .unexpected harm that occurs as a result of treatment or care, not directly because of a patient's illness or underlying condition." [31, p. 74] Using epidemiological estimates of national rates of iatrogenic injury, the study noted that approximately 44 to 66 serious iatrogenic injuries occur per 10,000 hospital admissions in the United States. Yet:

- Only two hospitals of more than 200 surveyed in the quoted study reported their rates of iatrogenic injury as within that range
- Half of the hospitals reported making fewer than five disclosures per 10,000 annual admissions
- The overall mean of disclosures per 10,000 annual admissions was 7.4, suggesting that if the scientific estimate of national rates of iatrogenic injury is correct, *these hospitals were disclosing only 10 to 20 percent of the serious, preventable, iatrogenic harms that occurred to their patients.*

As already noted, the health professional who realizes that his or her patient was harmed by a medical error has only three options: He or she can intentionally deceive the harmed party by way of concealment or a lie; he or she can disclose the error in a truthful and morally upright way; or he or she can alter or "edit" the disclosure—such as Finkelstein and his colleagues describe—in a way that perhaps tells the truth but is less than entirely truthful. The data currently suggest that the last option is probably the one most frequently employed by health professionals. A recent study on patients' and physicians' attitudes regarding the disclosure of medical errors found, "Many physicians spoke of 'choosing their words carefully' when talking with patients about errors. Most often, this careful choice of words involved mentioning the adverse event but not explicitly stating that an error took place." [32, p. 1004] This seemed especially the case in instances where the error might not be obvious, such as in administering the wrong medication (or the right medicine but the wrong dosage, route, mixed with the wrong diluent, etc.).

An excellent example of "choosing one's words carefully" was provided to me by the principal author of the just-mentioned study, Thomas Gallagher, who together with Wendy Levinson produced a training videotape on emotionally painful communications. Their tape on disclosing medical error, whose content they fashioned from interviews with practicing physicians, presents a physician entering a patient's room to explain why the patient had become unconscious and was transferred to the intensive care unit earlier that day.[33] The patient, Mr. Thompson, has fully recovered but the physician very much resists telling him the unadulterated truth, which is that the 100-unit insulin dose he received that morning constituted a ten-fold error over the 10-unit dose that she, his physician, had ordered the evening before. Her handwriting, however, was sloppy in that her "u" for units looked like a "0," and the unit clerk, nurse, and everyone else, misread or did not question the 100-unit order. When the physician enters Mr. Thompson's room, they exchange greetings, and the following conversation ensues:

Physician: Actually, I wanted to talk with you a bit more about what happened this morning and why you had to go the intensive care unit. As you know, people with diabetes can have wide swings in their blood sugar. This morning your blood sugar dropped all the way down to 35, which was dangerously low. This is why you passed out. Now, fortunately, we were able to get your blood sugar back up to a normal range so I anticipate things to go smoothly from here on out.

Mr. Thompson: That's sort of odd. My blood sugar has never been that low before. What do you think caused my blood sugar to be so low?

Physician: I'm almost positive it was a bad reaction to the insulin you got this morning. Now, we have adjusted your dose somewhat so this probably won't be a problem in the future.

Mr. Thompson (looking puzzled and slightly irritated): Bad reaction? What do you mean a bad reaction?

Physician: Looking back at your chart, it appears that you got more insulin than you needed. Now we have a better sense of how much insulin you require so that isn't likely to happen again.

Mr. Thompson (looking very puzzled): I've been on the same dose of insulin for the last four years. Exactly how much insulin did I get this morning?

Physician (nervously): It appears the nurse gave you 100 units of insulin rather than the 10 units you normally take. Apparently there was some kind of miscommunication about what your normal dose was.

Mr. Thompson (now very angry): What? 100 units? You're kidding me!! What kind of a moron would give a patient who usually gets 10 units of insulin a hundred units? Well, that could have killed me!!

Physician (chidingly): I understand why you're angry Mr. Thompson, but there's no need to yell.

Mr. Thompson (screaming): You'd be yelling too if someone almost killed you! Do you people have any idea of what you're doing here?

Physician (imploringly): The good news is that the episode that happened this morning isn't going to cause you permanent harm. Now, occasionally things like this do happen in the hospital much as we try to avoid them and prevent them. But what I would really like for us to do, Mr. Thompson, is work together and focus on moving forward and getting your emphysema under control so that you can go home from the hospital.

Notice how the physician cleverly conveys only the minimum of information at each exchange, but because the patient is aggressive with his questioning, the physician uncomfortably finds herself admitting more and more as the dialogue continues. Never does she say the words "error" or "mistake" nor does she mention her poor handwriting. Indeed her statements imply that the incident was either Mr. Thompson's fault—"People with diabetes have wide swings in their blood sugar . . . and your blood sugar dropped all the way down to 35."—or the nurse's fault—"It appears the nurse gave you 100 units of insulin rather than the 10 units you normally take." In any event, the physician says that the healthcare team saved the day for Mr. Thompson: "We were able to get your blood sugar back up to a normal range." Once Mr. Thompson learns of the error and becomes angry, the physician chides him for his anger and then tries to distract him with "the good news is … " Her refusal to make an effort to understand how Mr. Thompson is experiencing this situation is not atypical. She normalizes the error by saying, "These things happen," then asks Mr. Thompson to "work together" with her and the staff—implying that somehow he violated their partnership agreement—and then asks Mr. Thompson to forget the whole thing and "focus on moving forward." These maneuvers will be much discussed in what follows because they represent the physician's anxious insistence that Mr. Thompson *redirect his attention from the adverse event to what she finds comforting and salient about what happened*: namely, that the error did not cause permanent harm, that his insulin management should be fine from here on out, and what really merits clinical attention is his emphysema.

Mr. Thompson's increasing irritation as this conversation ensues is perfectly understandable. He is appalled at how this error is being minimized by the physician who cannot see beyond her own fears and psychological needs so as to attend to Mr. Thompson's, which are to 1) find out what really happened, 2) receive affirmation that the error ought not have occurred, and 3) have his feelings of outrage confirmed by the physician. Somehow, all the training this physician has received about patient-centered care and patient-centered ideals evaporated under a blanket of fear and a need to preserve her feelings of adequacy and competence.

In fact, health professionals such as this physician are known to be immensely clever at covering up or drawing attention away from an error by the language they use. There is good reason to believe their facility with linguistic subterfuge is cultivated during their residency years or specialty training. Fred Rosner and his colleagues remarked how "Admission of errors is difficult for physicians. Historically, physicians in residency have trained in a culture where disclosure to peers is a sign of weakness. Instead, skill in 'roundsmanship' is valued, that is, creative and contemporaneous responses to cover deficiencies or errors when reporting to more senior physicians."[34, p. 2090]

The remainder of this chapter explores the dimensions of "roundsmanship" and especially focuses on its moral ramifications. First, the discussion will examine the hypothesis that many health professionals, when faced with the fact that they committed a serious harm-causing error—such as in the example of Mr. Thompson—will strongly consider and often succumb to the temptation to rationalize the error or its concealment. Doing so enables those health providers who proceed with less than truthful disclosures to believe that their concealment or deception is *not* immoral. Then the discussion will advance the first elements of a model of narcissism as an explanatory paradigm for understanding the psychological roots of error rationalization and concealment.

Rationalizing the Concealment of Medical Error: Two Explanatory Models

Model No. 1: Resolving Cognitive Dissonance

In his best-selling 2002 book *Complications*, surgeon Atul Gawande noted that:

> When things go wrong, it's almost impossible for a physician to talk to a patient honestly about mistakes. Hospital lawyers warn doctors that, although they must, of course, tell patients about injuries that occur, they are never to intimate that they were at fault, lest the 'confession' wind up in court as damning evidence in a black-and-white morality tale. At most, a doctor might say, 'I'm sorry that things didn't go as well as we had hoped.'[35, p. 57]

Nearly 20 years earlier, though, physician David Hilfiker sounded a different, more psychologically oriented explanation for the physician's reluctance to disclose error truthfully and comprehensively:

> [I]t is almost impossible for practicing physicians to deal with their errors in a psychologically healthy fashion. . . . The climate of medical school and residency training, for instance, makes it nearly impossible to confront the emotional consequences of mistakes . . . "This is the mistake I made; I'm sorry." How can one say that to a grieving mother, to a family that has lost a member? It simply doesn't fit into the physician-patient relationship . . . Little wonder that physicians are accused of having a God complex; little wonder that we are defensive about our judgments; little wonder that we blame the patient or the previous physician when things go wrong, that we yell at the nurses for their mistakes.[36, p. 121]

Although no studies on the rationalization of medical error have as yet appeared, Hilfiker's suggestion that a process of rationalization or blame-shifting sometimes occurs among health professionals who commit error can be tested. Consequently, we undertook a modest survey of health professionals' beliefs on the frequency of error rationalization. The reasons for conducting this survey were to ascertain how common risk management professionals believe rationalizations of medical error are and whether such rationalizations adversely affect the degree to which medical errors are reported to hospital administration and are communicated to harmed parties. The three-question survey reproduced here was distributed over a number of months in 2002 to registrants at four hospital risk management conferences occurring in Dallas (TX), Kansas City (KS), Richmond (VA), and Columbus (OH). Respondents were primarily physicians, nurses, pharmacists, and quality assurance personnel, all of whom were professionally involved in patient safety operations at their hospitals and thus were well positioned to have a credible opinion on the nature and frequency of error rationalization. The survey was distributed and completed before respondents heard any conference presentations on error disclosure, so that they would not be influenced by any comments from program faculty on error concealment and its possible causes.

The findings indicate that audience members overwhelmingly agreed that error rationalization is common and that it profoundly inhibits error reporting and its subsequent disclosure to harmed parties.

RATIONALIZATION OF HARM-CAUSING ERROR SURVEY

Anecdotal evidence suggests that health providers sometimes "rationalize" their harm-causing medical errors. In other words, they use excuses such as the following to lessen the impact of the error, and to excuse themselves from having to report the error or disclose the error to the harmed patient or family. Some rationalizations that have been noted are:

"Why disclose the error? The patient was going to die anyway."

"Telling the family about this error will only make them feel worse."

"It was the patient's fault. If he wasn't so (obese, sick, etc.), this error wouldn't have caused so much harm."

"Well, we did our best. These things happen."

"If we're not totally and absolutely certain the error caused the harm, we don't have to tell."

The problem is there's no research on how common these rationalizations are. We are interested in your experience regarding error rationalizations. Please circle your degree of agreement or disagreement for each of the following statements.

N = 186

1. Rationalizations that excuse medical errors (and that excuse the need to disclose and report those errors) are common in hospitals.

Strongly Disagree	Disagree	Not Sure	Agree	Strongly Agree
1% (1)	7% (13)	4% (8)	62% (115)	26% (49)

2. Rationalizations are one of the chief reasons why errors are not reported or disclosed.

Strongly Disagree	Disagree	Not Sure	Agree	Strongly Agree
1% (1)	13% (24)	10% (18)	59% (111)	17% (32)

3. Healthcare providers are strongly tempted to rationalize their errors.

Strongly Disagree	Disagree	Not Sure	Agree	Strongly Agree
1% (1)	4% (7)	6% (12)	57% (106)	32% (60)

Now, while the fear of a malpractice suit subsequent to disclosure can indeed be the primary motivator for concealing an error, it does not entirely explain the phenomenon of rationalization. Jo-Ann Tsang characterized moral rationalization as "The cognitive process that individuals use to convince themselves that their behavior does not violate their moral standards."[37, p. 26] Make one addition to this: Moral rationalization is characterized by a weaker argument defeating a stronger one. The point is that a rationalizer will adopt a distorted or confabulated interpretation of an event because *that interpretation and whatever action plan it encourages relieves anxiety and confirms his or her self-understanding as that of a moral individual.*

Self-deception is key to an authentic rationalization. The health professional who explicitly realizes he or she conceals an error so as to avert a malpractice suit is too aware of his or her real motivations and does not succumb, by definition, to rationalization. If he or she deceives the patient through a dissimulation, the professional will know that he or she has lied, which might well compound his or her misery. In Christensen's study, one obviously non-rationalizing physician confessed, "I think the big issue for me is that nobody can absolve you. You recognize that everything you think is very self-serving and biased, so you can't rationalize your way out of it." [38, p. 426]

However, professionals who are successful rationalizers unconsciously succumb to their need to relieve the painful cognitive dissonances arising from, 1) wanting to sustain their identity and self-esteem as decent and moral professionals, with 2) the very unsettling fact that they committed a serious harm-causing error and that, 3) the right thing to do is disclose it to the harmed party. Acknowledging the error and the moral requirement of disclosure triggers immense psychological discomfort: On the one hand, the professional has a psychological need to sustain his or her self-image as a professionally competent and moral individual who does the right thing regardless of the consequences. On the other hand, the self-image of the technically competent and morally decent health professional might already have been assaulted by the commission of the error itself since many health professionals (wrongly) believe that the commission of error denotes a flawed character. Additionally, the professional is now contemplating a discussion with the harmed party that might put his or her personal and professional welfare at grave risk.

The objective of rationalization, then, is for the professional to convince him- or herself that error concealment (or a dissimulating disclosure) is not morally or professionally wrong. The rationalizer wants to be convinced of the rightness of his or her concealment or dissimulation because moral people do not violate ethical obligations connected with veracity, honesty, informed consent, or any other moral norms associated with the fiduciary nature of the professional-patient relationship. We will now turn to how this is accomplished.

How to Rationalize

The psychological objective of the rationalization is to *reinterpret* the moral situation—in this case, either the error scenario itself or a less-than-truthful communication of it to the harmed party—such that what would normally appear to be a deception becomes understood as morally acceptable. Psychologists have enumerated a variety of strategies whereby these reinterpretations might occur. Here are a few that Tsang mentions in her review of moral rationalization, that can be readily applied to harm-causing error scenarios:[39]

- *Euphemistic language.* Here, words and phrases are carefully chosen such that the immoral act is seen as harmless. Thus, the error discloser might refer to the harm-causing error and its aftermath as a "complication," "medical misadventure," or "incident." A blatant failure to spot a lesion on an X-ray becomes translated as "an unappreciated lesion." A malpractice case, which shall be discussed more elaborately in Chapter 4, involved a woman who sustained global anoxia, apparently as a result of an anesthesiologist's failure to restart the ventilator after he had intentionally turned it off to permit the surgeon to take an X-ray of the patient's abdomen. In explaining the incident to the woman's family, the surgeon reiterated the patient's having had a "stroke" while the anesthesiologist initially kept reiterating to the surgeon that "she was off the vent," making it somehow sound as though it was the patient's fault. With enough repetition, the health professional might convince him- or herself that these phrases are entirely accurate accounts of what happened.

- *Advantageous comparison.* Here, the individual rationalizes concealment by comparing it to something worse. Thus a commonly heard error concealment rationalization used by health professionals is, "Telling the family will only make them feel worse than they already do." Essential to this rationalization is the confabulation necessary to make the immoral act *advantageously* compare to—and thus trump—the moral act. Indeed, this example uses certain elements of the next rationalization technique.

- *Distorting the consequences of an action.* Here, guilt avoidance occurs by the professional's reinterpretation of what happened and its likely aftermath. The attraction of this rationalization consists in its relieving the obligation to disclose, because the harm the error caused has been transformed into something non-harmful, even beneficial. A lethal error, for example, can become a "blessing in disguise" or "a valuable learning experience." The health professional convinces himself that, "Telling the family will only make them feel worse than they already do," although it is well known that harmed parties are infuriated and feel betrayed when they discover that error was concealed from them.

- *Displacement of responsibility.* Here, the individual pleads that what seemed to be his or her immoral act was actually caused by someone else who is really to blame.

Thus the professional who is reluctant to disclose error in a truthful or comprehensive way can blame the insurance carrier whose malpractice policy forbids an admission of liability.

- *Diffusion of responsibility.* Here, the individual transfers responsibility for what happened to others or to the group as a whole. Thus, responsibility for a medication error can be spread to any number of persons (e.g., the physician who writes the order, the unit clerk who transcribes it, the nurse who checks the transcription, the pharmacist who fills it, and the nurses who check, recheck, and administer the medication). Although one person in this continuum might be the "salient" error operator, it can be argued that each one is equally to blame for whatever harm the patient sustained. By fragmenting and dispersing the error to the entire group, its harmfulness becomes no one's primary fault.

- *Attributions of blame.* A common example of blame attribution is when the perpetrator blames the victim or the circumstances for enabling the harm to occur. Thus, women are blamed for their being raped. Or to use a completely different example, an overemphasis on quarterly earnings might be blamed for the overly aggressive accounting practices that ultimately lead to the downfall of a large corporation. In error scenarios, it is not uncommon to blame the patient for the error, as in "Had the patient taken better care of himself, the harm he sustained wouldn't have been so bad." Indeed, the next chapter offers an historical example of Sigmund Freud's blaming a patient for an embarrassing, error-caused outcome.

- *Fragmentation.* Here, the individual fragments or "splits" him- or herself so that attention can be diverted from the "bad self" who might have done something morally problematic to the good and more fundamental self who continues to be concerned about the welfare of others. Holocaust scholars note that concentration camp guards sometimes wrote heartfelt letters home, inquiring about the welfare of their wives and children—perhaps as a way of reassuring themselves of their humanity and goodness. Delivering healthcare, of course, confirms the health professional's abiding goodness. Thus, the physician who commits a horrendous error in the morning but saves two lives in the afternoon might convince herself of her basic goodness and excuse the error and its concealment as aberrations.

Note that in all of this, rationalization is used both to affirm one's self-concept as a good and decent person and to ward off extremely upsetting feelings of guilt and anxiety for engaging in acts that would otherwise count as deceitful or immoral. Rationalization, then, is triggered by the professional's narcissistically based need to maintain his or her self-esteem. This line of argument continues in the next section where the explanatory model looks to the brain's exquisite architecture and its inherent interest in survival to explain the phenomenon of moral rationalization in concealing medical error.

Model No. 2: Daniel Goleman's Model of Moral Attentiveness

It is interesting to note a uniform phenomenon in the various forms of rationalization previously described. Each one *diverts attention* from the primary moral obligation at stake, namely error disclosure, toward a different course of action that turns out to be more appealing because it is more comforting. For example, rationalizing on the basis of "advantageous comparison" effectively says: "Think of how doing the seemingly correct thing, that is, disclosing the error, will only make everyone worse off. Now, how can that be the 'right' thing? Granted, the situation as it stands now is less than ideal, but leaving it that way is really the best option when you consider what might result from doing what others would tell you is morally 'right.'" Rationalization enables error concealment or dissimulation to "feel" better. It enables the moral dilemma to be shorn of its discomfort so that it ceases to be a dilemma. Consequently—and here is the pay-off—the more a person entertains and buys into the rationalization, the better he or she feels.

In his book *Vital Lies, Simple Truths,* Daniel Goleman offers a provocative explanation of rationalization that uses a kind of bioevolutionary model and that can be applied in a remarkably illuminating way to rationalizing the concealment of medical error.[40] The centerpiece of Goleman's hypothesis consists in how rationalization diverts a sense of moral *attentiveness* away from an uncomfortable but nevertheless morally right course of action toward a morally problematic option that nevertheless feels much more comfortable.

Goleman begins by noting how fundamental, survival-oriented forms of attention (e.g., becoming hyperalert if crossing paths with a rattlesnake) are neurobiologically based. In situations wherein the sense of survival is threatened, the body registers a stress response so that the brain's hypothalamus, pituitary, and adrenal glands release various neurotransmitters and hormones that physiologically enable a person to better cope with the threat. During instances wherein a person is physically attacked or threatened, the brain will trigger, among other things, a rush of endorphins, opioids, and a hormone acronymized to ACTH (for adrencorticotrophic hormone). ACTH is released into the bloodstream but returns to the brain and acts on the adrenal cortex and glands to signal the release of epinephrine and glucocorticoids into the bloodstream that prepare the body's muscle, heart, and lungs for a fight or flight response.[41]

At first glance, the conjunctive release of endorphins with ACTH is exceedingly odd because endorphins both ease pain and lessen a person's attention. ACTH heightens attention and appears to increase sensitivity to pain. Researchers have found, however, that ACTH streams into and has its pain-sensitizing and thus attentional effect on the body first, whereupon the endorphins have their pain dulling effects seconds or minutes later. Consequently, the brain's first response of pain alerts an individual to the danger, while the brain's second response diminishes the pain he or she might feel from it. Bioevolutionists speculate that the reason for this neuromodulatory two-step is to alert the organism, first, that it is in very serious trouble but then to diminish the way physical pain might compromise the organism's survival opportunities through immobilizing fear or panic.[42]

Goleman suggests that this model might have direct explanatory application to the psychological role of attention in stressful situations. While immediate attention to the threat is paramount in surviving (e.g., the mouse who is indifferent to being attacked by a cat is as good as dead), the organism's inability to shift attention to something other than its pain—i.e., to a flight or fight response—would spell its doom. The brain therefore initially alerts the organism with an unambiguous pain sensation to attend to the danger and then redirects attention to various survival options. The fact that the brain has evolved this strategy over millions of years attests to its success. Moreover, the human nervous system's first alert is a narcissistically, "me-oriented" one: Protect yourself. This kind of hard-wiring is impossible to overcome, unless the neural pathways are surgically or traumatically affected or one performs meditation or cognitive exercises such that he or she becomes indifferent to survival.

ATTENTION AND STRESS

Given their descriptions, it is clear that the health professionals mentioned at the beginning of the chapter experienced an immensely unpleasant stress response to their realization that they committed a serious error. But recall that these professionals not only understood their stress to be about the patient's welfare, but about their own welfare as well. It is hardly a stretch to hypothesize that under such conditions, where a person feels his or her own welfare to be at stake, the brain will search for a strategy that can ameliorate this psychological trauma. Goleman notes that:

> While stress arousal is a fitting mode to meet emergency, as an ongoing state it is a disaster. Sustained stress arousal leads to pathology: anxiety states or psychosomatic disorders such as hypertension. These diseases are end products of the stress response, the cost of an unrelenting readiness for emergency.
>
> That response is in reaction to the perception of threat. Tuning out threat is one way to short-circuit stress arousal. Indeed for those dangers and pains that are mental, selective attention offers relief. Denial is the psychological analogue of the endorphin attentional tune-out.[43, p. 43]

In 2002, Mark Ellenbogen and his colleagues at Concordia and McGill Universities published the results of a series of experiments that corroborated Goleman's hypothesis that stressful situations will encourage a person's attention to shift away from unpleasant thoughts toward more calming ones.[44] After inducing stress in their subjects, the researchers then flashed a series of emotionally pleasant, unpleasant, and neutral words on a computer screen. They found that research participants who were experimentally induced to have stress rapidly disengaged their attention from negative words (e.g., "misery," "ruined," "useless," "failure," "inferior," "helpless," "disaster," "disgrace") but not from neutral or positive ones (e.g., "success," "strong," "talented"). This finding led the research team to hypothesize, "Perhaps, participants in the present study attempted to terminate an emotional response to repetitive loss (i.e., the stressful situation) by avoiding negative stimuli. Thus prolonged exposure to an emotional cue may initiate intentional responses to self-regulate by way of attentional avoidance."[45, p.729] Furthermore and of considerable importance to this study on error, the study's participants who reported varying but notable levels of depression were found to have marked *slowness* in disengaging attention from any of the words. This led to the speculation, "Perhaps, slow attentional disengagement precipitates maladaptive coping strategies such as excessive perseveration or rumination on negative themes."[46, p.730] In terms of error commission, this implies that health professionals who already experience some form of depression are at serious psychological risk from the emotional trauma of error realization. They may ultimately find themselves unable to disengage their attention from the horror of the event, and they might become a serious risk to themselves or others.

This experiment speaks to Goleman's model that targets selective or biased attention as a medium of denial in explaining rationalization. As the organism is biologically disposed to extinguish its painful stimuli, so it attends to and cultivates something that might work as a mechanism of relief. In moral situations, if the factual and/or moral reality of the event is too painful to acknowledge and its appropriate moral resolution even more painful, the event can be reconstructed through rationalization so that a person's sense of moral salience (i.e., what ought to be done or how to understand what is happening) is redefined. Ultimately, rationalization is a kind of moral counterfeit such that a moral lapse, which in this case is error concealment, becomes morally acceptable.

Application of the Selective Attention Model to Concealing Medical Error

Goleman's model is interesting because of how he emphasizes the role of "selective" attention in re-conceptualizing and re-interpreting the event. Specifically, the organism *selectively attends to some feature of the threat situation and then uses that feature to concoct a rationalization*—as in the examples that Tsang supplied—whereby the extremely unpleasant feelings triggered by the threat situation are eliminated. This selective attentiveness to some situational aspect implies an *inattentiveness to* or denial of other contextual aspects which are, of course, the morally obligatory but psychologically painful ones.

The phenomenon of error rationalization is impressively explained by Goleman's model. For example, a physician at a medical conference was heard challenging the very idea of disclosing error by asserting that medical experts often disagree about whether or not "X" was an error. "So, how can you expect practitioners to disclose errors when not even the experts agree on what error is?" he asked. Goleman's model immediately points out how that individual conveniently shifted his attention from countless examples that everyone would agree are errors, such as wrong side or wrong patient surgeries. By asking the audience members to fix their attention on a particular aspect of the comprehensive phenomenon of medical error—namely, that experts occasionally disagree on whether a discrete instance of medical judgment or behavior qualifies as an error—this individual seeks to dismiss *entirely* the validity of error disclosure and the psychological discomfort it arouses. Important to note is that members of the audience who agreed with the physician also shared in his moral inattentiveness.

Goleman's model posits a "selection-reinterpretation" phenomenon whereby some situational aspect or contour is lifted from the situational whole—and to the exclusion or denial of more morally weighty situational elements—and then heavily imbued or injected with moral salience by way of an imaginative reconstruction/distortion of the event. One form of this selection-reinterpretation process in error concealment rationalizations consists in the professional's attending to a *causal or before-the-harm* feature of the error sequence. In these instances, there is no disagreement over the fact that an adverse outcome eventually occurred; instead, what is denied or dismissed is that the health professional caused the harm. Consider the following examples, which are inspired by actual cases:

- Immediately following surgery, a tube draining fluid from the patient's chest is mistakenly connected to a continuous suction pump. The pump creates an inordinately high degree of negative pressure in the patient's chest, and it dislodges the sutures the surgeon placed in the patient's pulmonary artery. The surgical team is unable to stop the bleeding and the patient dies. The surgeon tells the family that their loved one "began to bleed as a result of the operation" and that, "although every effort was made to stop the bleeding," the patient did not survive. The operating room team contends that the "truth was told," but they do not disclose the error to the family because the health professional who deployed the continuous suction pump by mistake had never before assisted at that particular type of surgery. Because her inexperience was not her fault and because "the possibility of hemorrhage" was mentioned in the informed consent process, error concealment was rationalized.

- Nurse Jones is assigned to an extremely busy patient care unit at which she had never worked. When she replaces an IV bag, she sets the IV pump at an incorrect flow rate, resulting in a massive fluid overdose for the patient. The patient then requires transfer to the intensive care unit for treatment for acute congestive heart failure and nearly dies. It is decided not to disclose this error to the patient because the "real" causes of the error—not enough staff, overly stressed and burned out nursing personnel, "floating" of inexperienced staff from other units—is a system problem that is beyond the control, and therefore beyond the responsibility, of the nursing staff.

- Before ordering an antibiotic, Dr. Jones asks the patient if he has any allergies to antibiotics. The patient stares blankly at Dr. Jones for a moment and then answers, "No." The patient's allergy to antibiotics, however, is conspicuously noted on his medical record, which Dr. Jones fails to read carefully. Less than an hour after receiving the drug, the patient experiences aching joints, a headache, and a skin rash. Although the drug allergy is later noted, rather than admit that an error occurred because of a careless reading of the patient's medical record, Dr. Jones admonishes the patient for failure to know about his drug allergy and to alert the staff to it.

- A patient who has just had a stroke is admitted to hospital and by mistake receives twice the dosage of a drug that he was supposed to receive to control seizures. The drug is known to cause respiratory depression. He subsequently has a cardio-respiratory arrest and dies. The family is told that the patient might have had an adverse drug reaction but they are not told about the error because, "We cannot say for certain that the incorrect dosage caused his arrest."

In each of these cases, attention is diverted from either the erring professional or his or her mistake and profoundly away from the patient's right to know about the error and toward another element in the causal or before-harm sequence of affairs that can be reformulated into a justification for concealment. The rationalizers in the first scenario, for example, neither question the moral propriety of assigning an unskilled operating room nurse to a complex operation, nor do they reflect on the remarkable equivocation of the term "possibility of hemorrhage" as resulting from either a negligent or non-negligent act.

However, another type of rationalization using selective attention occurs when *the outcome or the consequence of the error is confabulated.* Unlike the above, these instances do not deny the fault of the error operator. Rather they deny that a serious harm resulted or that disclosure would be beneficial to the affected parties. Consider the following two examples:

- Surgeon Smith does a wrong-side carotid endarterectomy on Mr. Harris. Although both of Mr. Harris's carotid arteries are blocked and need surgery, the right is more blocked than the left and so is the one scheduled for operation. Midway through the procedure, which is otherwise uneventful, Dr. Smith realizes he's operating on the left, non-consented artery. He finishes the surgery and approaches Mrs. Harris, who is in the waiting room. Dr. Smith smiles broadly and says to her, "The surgery went great. Now, although the paperwork reflected the right side, we went ahead and did the left side instead. Your husband's doing fine, and we'll do the right side in a few weeks." Mrs. Harris is somewhat bewildered but smiles and nods agreeably. The physician later declares that he acted in a perfectly professional fashion by telling Mrs. Harris the truth and that because both of Mr. Harris's arteries needed surgery, whichever one got surgically unblocked first was relatively unimportant.

- A terminally ill patient who is apparently in her final days of life is admitted to a hospital. A prescription is written for 10 milligrams of oxycodone, but she is given 100 milligrams by mistake and dies within an hour. The decision is made to say only that she might have had a bad reaction to some medicine she was receiving because, "The patient was going to die anyway, and our mistake didn't change anything." Further discussion of whether or not to tell the family of the medication error elicits the suggestions that, "telling the family will only make them feel worse" and that given the patient's condition, perhaps the error should be understood as a "blessing in disguise."

Whether the rationalization denies the error, the error operator's culpability, or the gravity of the outcome, it is important to point out that "lacunose" attentional patterns can and do become adopted by an entire group. Whatever elements of the clinical scenario the group decides merit attention versus the ones to which they are morally inattentive require an interpretational framework that the entire group adopts. Moral inattentiveness therefore admits a cognitional conspiracy.

Conclusion: Is Rationalization Conscious or Not?

By way of concluding this chapter, consider whether the rationalization patterns discussed above are consciously constructed or not. Assuming that the question inquires about whether or not the rationalizer is aware of the real, underlying motivation of his rationalization, contemporary neurophilosophers might propose the following explanation: Moral learning largely occurs from socialization, and moral concepts are learned not through philosophical intellectualization but through experience. This means that not only are concepts such as honesty mediated by the society in which exposure to honesty occurs, it also means that moral concepts are learned with all the untidiness and experiential richness that real-world situations display.[47]

   Neuroethicists suggest that the constitutive features of moral constructs (or representations) are learned through countless experiences with real-life contexts wherein those constructs are "absorbed" by the brain's neural pathways or neural "nets."[48] For example, the neural assemblage for "truth telling" that develops in the brain is a cluster of neural channels that mediate the comprehension and management of situations in which veracity is at issue. This assemblage of brain materials admits a prototypical pattern of activation or what is also called a "central tendency"—a fundamental cognitive-behavioral disposition such as "tell the truth"—that is triggered if the situation at hand has features that are similar to those centrally embedded in the prototype that has evolved in the brain. Of course, the prototype or central tendency will also be triggered by cases wherein truth telling might be problematic. This is how morality is learned and one's moral sense is refined. Under this neurological model, moral situations are problematic when their constitutive features simultaneously share certain strong elemental features with the prototype but depart from the prototype with equally strong but vastly different features.[49]

For example, assume that upon nearly finishing a surgery, a physician has an X-ray taken to ensure that no surgical artifacts remain inside the patient. The X-ray reveals a small, radio-opaque piece of gauze called a pledget, which the surgeon, by re-opening a few sutures, easily removes. Another X-ray is taken and reveals nothing unusual. The surgery is then completed and the patient does fine. If the hospital has an error disclosure policy, ought the patient be told of the pledget incident? While it was an error, it was quickly discerned, removed without incident, and caused no harm. But the recovery of the pledget was nevertheless noted in the patient's surgical record so the patient or a family member might learn about it and ask if it constituted a mistake. Moreover, if instead of the procedure's requiring a few minutes to remove the pledget, suppose 45 minutes were required. Would the additional time the patient needed to be anesthetized have argued for the error being more serious and therefore have more strongly argued for disclosure? This case illustrates how the "proximity" of an incident with the brain's "error disclosure prototype" will affect one's moral sense. The more proximate or the more the incident's elements mesh with the prototype, the more one will feel a moral obligation as dictated by the prototype. The less the representation's constitutive elements have in common with the prototype, the less inclined the individual will be to disclose.

On this neurological account, the error rationalizer will try to de-emphasize precisely those elements of the real-life scenario that argue for disclosure, that is, are proximate to the prototype—while accentuating the ones that don't. Now, the more reflexive, automatic, and immediate is the individual's adverting to and adopting rationalization, the more his or her rationalization seems to occur below the horizon of awareness. This is because such reflexivity indicates the brain's ready capitulation to the largely unconscious fears of dire consequences eventuating from disclosure, or from an intensely conditioned, largely unreflective, and therefore mostly unconscious ascription of contextual meanings that incline one toward moral cowardice. On the other hand, the more the individual evinces a struggle between his or her self-serving impulses that encourage error rationalization versus considerations about what the patient is owed, as articulated in section 8.12 of the AMA code, the more conscientious and attentive he or she will be of various competing motives and reasons to rationalize. If this individual has neural representations that are strongly supported by "moral emotions" that incline him or her to ethical, other-regarding behavior despite the pain he or she may nevertheless experience by owning the error, he or she will be said to be morally courageous.

Unfortunately though, this explanation has a rather tautologous ring. It basically says: People who rationalize successfully are unconscious of it because the unconscious part of their brain overwhelms the conscious part. Whereas people who do not succumb to rationalization have brain activity whose "ethical" prominences can somehow withstand and discern the unconscious rationalizing inclinations that otherwise characterize more primitive, less ethically aware brain activity. These latter individuals enjoy "ethical" neural contents and are able to bring their ethical emotions into play because they possess a kind of brain activity that rationalizers either have not developed or have repressed.

While this may well be a tautology, it is certainly the case that some individuals, upon being shown that they have engaged in rationalization, will admit it without much resistance. For them, the real motive for rationalization was on the cusp of their conscious awareness so that someone's exposing the rationalization as a rationalization elicits what the former dimly recognized but found too painful to acknowledge. On the other hand, there will doubtlessly be those individuals who accept rationalization categorically and who stoutly deny that their moral sensibilities are clouded by the self-serving objectives that rationalization offers. For them, the semantic content of their rationalization is ethically persuasive because they cannot (or refuse to) discern how its palliative effect obliterates their moral sense. Their unconscious has enabled the very objective that rationalization provides: to convert an immoral act into a moral one that sustains their self-image as a moral person.

As an ending to this chapter, recall one of its observations: Individuals will use their self-formations in recruiting management strategies for moral dilemmas. The next chapter will build on the role of the "self" in reacting to medical error by examining a frankly troubling aspect about the moral selves of some health providers—namely, their penchant for narcissistically inclined behaviors. This chapter has hinted at a neuropsychological model of narcissism in terms of the self-protective reflexes that health professionals inevitably experience in the face of a threat to their welfare, as in disclosing a medical error. The next chapter offers a psychoanalytical account of narcissism and will argue that a narcissistic self-formation is a primary reason for not only self-serving responses to medical error, but for responses that lack empathy for patients in general. The commission of a medical error will be depicted in the next chapter as a narcissistic outrage that, in conjunction with the brain activity described in this chapter, continues to compromise a patient-centered response.

References

1. Govier, Trudy. *Forgiveness and Revenge.* New York: Routledge, 2002.
2. Wolf, Zane Robinson. *Medication Errors: The Nursing Experience.* Albany, NY: Delmar Publishers, Inc., 1994.
3. Christensen, John F.; Levinson, Wendy; and Dunn, Patrick M. "The heart of darkness: The impact of perceived mistakes on physicians." *Journal of General Internal Medicine.* 7 (July/August):424–431, 1992.
4. Christensen et al., 1992.
5. Gallagher, Thomas H.; Waterman, Amy D.; Ebers, Alison G.; Fraser, Victoria J.; and Levinson, Wendy. "Patients' and physicians' attitudes regarding the disclosure of medical errors." *JAMA.* 289(8):1001–1007, 2003.

6. Joint Commission. *2002 Hospital Accreditation Standards.* Oakbrook Terrace, IL:Joint Commission, 2002.

7. Personal communication from Hal Bresslar, Joint Commission attorney.

8. Tansill, David. Disclosing unanticipated outcomes under JCAHO standard. (Medical Association of Georgia Mutual Insurance Company) *Healthcare Risk Manager.* 8(16):1–4, 2002.

9. American Institute for CPCU. *CPCU Handbook of Insurance Practices.* Malvern, PA: Insurance Institute of America, 1998.

10. The states thus far (3/2004) are Massachusetts, California, Florida, Texas, Washington, and Oregon. See respectively, Mass Gen. Laws, ch. 233, section 23 D; Cal. Evid. Code section 1160; Fla. Stat. Ann. Section 90.4026; Tex. Civ. Prac. & Rem. Code Ann. Section 18.0612; Wash. Rev. Code Ann. Section 5.66.010; 2003 Or. Laws Ch. 384 (H.B. 3361), approved June 16, 2003.

11. 2003 Colo. Legis. Serv. Ch. 126 (H.B. 03-1232), approved Apr. 17, 2003.

12. Council on Ethical and Judicial Affairs. *Code of Medical Ethics: Current Opinions with Annotations.* 2002–2003 Edition. Chicago, IL: AMA Press, 2002.

13. Witman, Amy B.; Park, Deric M.; and Hardin, Steven B. "How do patients want physicians to handle mistakes?" *Archives of Internal Medicine.* 156(Dec 9/23):2565–2569, 1996; Vincent, Charles; Young, Magi; and Phillips, Angela. "Why do people sue doctors?" *Lancet.* 343(8913):1609–1613, 1994; Hingorani, Melanie; Wong, Tina; and Vafidis, Gilli. "Patients' and doctors' attitudes to amount of information given after unintended injury during treatment: Cross-sectional, questionnaire survey." *British Medical Journal.* 318(7184):640–641, 1999.

14. University HealthSystem Consortium. *Shining the Light on Errors: How Open Should We Be?* Oak Brook, IL: University Health System Consortium, 2002.

15. Banja, John. "Disclosing medical error: How much to tell?" *Journal of Healthcare Risk Management.* 23(1):11–14, 2003.

16. Banja, 2003.

17. Banja, 2003.

18. Smith, Martin L., and Forster, Heidi P. "Morally managing medical mistakes." *Cambridge Quarterly of Healthcare Ethics.* 9(1):38–53, 2000.

19. Personal communication. Mr. Reezin N. Swilley, former assistant vice-president of human resources at BellSouth, Atlanta, GA. January 27, 2002.

20. "Disclosure of patient safety events." Available from Legal Services, Licking Memorial Health Systems, 1320 West Main Street, Newark, Ohio 43055.

21. King, Joseph. H. *The Law of Medical Malpractice in a Nutshell,* 2nd Edition. St. Paul, MN: West Publishing Company, 1986. pp. 39–43; Sage, William M.; Hastings, Kathleen E.; and Berenson, Robert A. "Enterprise liability for medical malpractice and healthcare quality improvement." *American Journal of*

Law and Medicine. 20:128, 1994; Bovbjerg, Randall R., and Sloan, Frank A. "No-fault for medical injury: theory and evidence." *University of Cincinnati Law Review.* 67(Fall):53423, 1998.

22. Witman, Park, and Hardin, 1996.

23. Perper, Joshua. "Life-threatening and fatal therapeutic misadventures." In *Human Error in Medicine*, Marilyn Sue Bogner, ed., Hillsdale, NJ: Lawrence Erlbaum Associates, 1994, pp. 2752.

24. Smith and Forster, 2000.

25. Finkelstein, Daniel; Wu, Albert W.; Holtzman, Neil A.; and Smith, Melanie K. "When a physician harms a patient by a medical error: Ethical, legal, and risk-management considerations." *The Journal of Clinical Ethics.* 8(4):330335, 1997.

26. Sweet, Matthew P., and Bernat, James L. "A study of the ethical duty of physicians to disclose errors." *The Journal of Clinical Ethics.* 8(4):341348, 1997.

27. Sweet and Bernat, 1997.

28. Sweet and Bernat, 1997.

29. Kohn, Linda T.; Corrigan, Janet M.; and Donaldson, Molla S. *To Err Is Human: Building a Safer Health System.* Washington, DC: National Academy Press, 2000.

30. Lamb, Rae M.; Studdert, David M.; Bohmer, Richard M. J.; Berwick, Donald M.; and Brennan, Troyen A. "Hospital disclosure practices: Results of a national survey." *Health Affairs.* 22(2):7383, 2003.

31. Lamb et al., 2003.

32. Gallagher et al., 2003.

33. *Discussing Tough Issues with Patients: Unreasonable Requests, Mistakes, Conflicts of Interest: Errors.* A videotape created by Thomas Gallagher, MD and Wendy Levinson, MD. Supported by a grant from the Network Program, Center for the Health Professions, University of California, San Francisco. Requests for information can be sent to Dr. Thomas Gallagher, University of Washington School of Medicine, 1959 NE Pacific St., Box 356178, Seattle, WA 981950001.

34. Rosner, Fred; Berger, Jeffrey T.; Kark, Pieter; Potash, Joel; and Bennett, Allen J.; for the Committee on Bioethical Issues of the Medical Society of the State of New York. "Disclosure and prevention of medical errors." *Archives of Internal Medicine.* 160(14):20892092.

35. Gawande, Atul. *Complications.* New York: Metropolitan Books, Henry Holt and Company, 2002.

36. Hilfiker, David. "Sounding board: Facing our mistakes." *New England Journal of Medicine.* 310(2):118422, 1984.

37. Tsang, Jo-Ann. "Moral rationalization and the integration of situational factors and psychological processes in immoral behavior." *Review of General Psychology*. 6(1):25–50, 2002.

38. Christensen et al., 1992.

39. Tsang, 2002.

40. Goleman, Daniel. *Vital Lies, Simple Truths: The Psychology of Self-Deception*. London, UK: Bloomsbury Publishing, 1997.

41. Goleman, 1997.

42. Goleman, 1997.

43. Goleman, 1997.

44. Ellenbogen, Mark A.; Schwartzman, Alexs E.; Stewart Jane; and Walker, Claire-Dominique. "Stress and selective attention: The interplay of mood, cortisol levels, and emotional information processing." *Psychophysiology*. 39: 723–732, 2002.

45. Ellenbogen et al., 2002.

46. Ellenbogen et al., 2002.

47. Flanagan, Owen. "The moral network," in *The Churchlands and Their Critics*, Robert N. McCauley, ed. Cambridge, MA: Blackwell Publishers, 1996, pp. 192–215.

48. Churchland, Paul M. *The Engine of Reason, the Seat of the Soul*. Cambridge, MA: MIT Press, 2000, pp. 143–150.

49. Churchland, 2000.

Chapter 3

Narcissism

"I pretended to be somebody I wanted to be and finally, I became that person. Or he became me."
Attributed to Cary Grant

"Reinhard was never his mother's favorite—and he was an only child."[1, item 749]
Thomas Berger

"Physicians are trained in narcissism."[2, p. 9]
Howard Spiro

"Physicians are often said to be narcissistic. No doubt some of them act in a way that has inspired the caricature of the vain, self-aggrandizing prima donna who assigns an intern the job of opening doors. But that is certainly not typical. The narcissism of most physicians is subtler."[3, p. 27]
Glen O. Gabbard and Roy Menninger

Introduction

The previous chapter suggests that considerations about patient-centered care and patient rights make up the moral fabric of medical error disclosure. The conscientious professional feels morally distressed if the patient's right to be informed about his or her care is disappointed. Consequently, we ought not be surprised if many health professionals are inclined to rationalize or confabulate their failure to disclose a harm-causing error as a way to diminish their guilt over its concealment, and because they are horrified at the prospects of a lawsuit as a result of their honesty. Rationalizing so that the nondisclosure of harm-causing error seems justified offers a health professional immense relief from the anxiety that error disclosure can arouse.

This chapter discusses a companion phenomenon to rationalization that is not uncommon in healthcare but that, like rationalization, also compromises the patient-centered sensibilities at the moral core of error disclosure. This is the phenomenon of narcissism which, because of its quintessentially self-regarding nature, denotes a psychological formation that is the antithesis of patient- or other-regarding behaviors. So as to head off hostile reactions to this chapter's theme at the outset, I must say that in no way am I asserting that the majority of health professionals are pathological narcissists. Indeed, pathological narcissism is fairly rare in the population at large while many healthcare professionals believe that there is a fully legitimate sense in talking about an emotionally "healthy" narcissist.[4] Rather, this chapter explores the hypothesis that there is an idiosyncratic kind of narcissist in healthcare, whom I will rather unimaginatively term a "medical narcissist." This medical narcissist is notable for 1) his or her lack of empathy for patients, 2) a compulsive and insistent treatment-oriented focus that winds up "subtracting" the patient from his or her disease, and 3) a communication/relational style that seeks to control the patient's beliefs, feelings, and actions. While the medical narcissist resorts to a host of narcissistic-like behaviors to control the therapeutic relationship, he or she is typically more psychologically healthy and emotionally well adjusted than his or her pathological counterpart. However, what inclines medical narcissists toward whatever degree of pathology they may exhibit is the way they use narcissistic-like behaviors to shore up a fragile self that needs protection from emotional anxiety and discomfort.

The following pages will show that:

- Not all narcissism is pathological.
- Any individual's narcissism is an amalgamation of healthy or unhealthy narcissistic traits, while any one of those traits can exist in a mild, moderate, or strong form.
- There are many varieties of narcissism that might be characterized on a continuum from very pathological to very healthy.
- Physicians as well as other health professionals do not typically evince the classical portrait of the pathological narcissist to any significant degree.
- Many physicians and other health professionals nevertheless demonstrate a kind of muted or closeted narcissism whose associated behaviors serve as a form of self-protection when their feelings of adequacy, control, or competency are threatened. Needless to say, the realization that they might have committed a medical error is a moment that can easily trigger these narcissistic defenses.

To begin, this chapter discusses and contrasts the healthy narcissist from his or her pathological counterpart, and then examines how a variant of the latter construct might manifest itself in healthcare. At that point, especially by way of characterizing how the medical narcissist is notable for his or her lack of empathy, compulsiveness, and rigidity, the chapter shows how that self-formation is poorly equipped to acknowledge or disclose harm-causing medical error in a patient-centered fashion. Perhaps the following discussion will make it much more obvious as to why certain health professionals, and especially many physicians, have difficulty not only in managing and disclosing medical error, but in managing any kind of activity that threatens their feelings of adequacy or competence.

Healthy and Pathological Narcissism

The Healthy Narcissist

In order to appreciate the psychological formation of the pathological narcissist, I will begin by examining his or her opposite formation, the healthy narcissist. While not all psychologists prefer the term "healthy narcissist," a number are keen to point out that not all narcissism is pathological. For example, James Masterson, a psychiatrist and leading authority on narcissistic character disorders, noted that, "[N]ormal, healthy narcissism is the capacity to identify what you want and need, get yourself together, and go after it, while also taking account of the welfare of others."[5, p. 94]

Prima facie, there is nothing pathological about feeling frustrated, angry, or depressed when life becomes difficult. Pathology occurs when a person becomes morbidly stuck in unproductive feelings and moods, or habitually responds to life's challenges in ways that fail to sustain healthy human relationships or that result in unhappiness or craziness. The physical therapist who catches herself blaming and feeling angry at a patient for his lack of therapeutic progress is acknowledging a narcissistically based vulnerability (i.e., her need to feel clinically competent by effecting a good functional outcome) but is hardly a narcissist on that account. On the other hand, the therapist who is easily frustrated by such patients; who cannot appreciate them as individuals with interests and beliefs different from hers; who understands them as the means by which she can prove herself to others; and who claims exclusive credit for each of her therapeutic successes but for none of her failures indeed fits the mold of an unhealthy narcissist.

In a series of studies appearing over the 1990s, Paul Watson and his colleagues at the University of Tennessee administered a battery of inventories and surveys that measure narcissistic traits to hundreds of college students, and then correlated the findings.[6] They concluded that the phenomenon of "healthy" narcissism is empirically verifiable in that persons with healthy self-esteem and reasonably good psychological adjustment can indeed score high on what would otherwise seem prototypically narcissistic traits, such as feelings of superiority, authority, perfection, self-absorption, self-admiration, and even arrogance. On the other hand, these very characteristics can also correlate with the decidedly pathological narcissist whose self-formation admits very poor adjustment, emotional exploitation, excessive hostility toward and envy of others, excessive demand for admiration, and deficient empathy. (See Figure 1 for a list of clinical characteristics that describe the narcissistic personality disorder.)

The decisive variable that distinguishes the healthy from the unhealthy narcissist appears to be healthy self-esteem.[7] Its presence or absence is crucial in determining whether assertiveness, self-absorption, or leadership aspirations correlate with a person who enjoys a sense of healthy pride and self-confidence, or whether they correlate with a person who is emotionally fragile, exploitative, and relentlessly intent on proving his or her worth to the world.

Figure 1 *DSM-IV traits for the narcissistic personality disorder**

- Grandiosity/ exaggerates achievements
- Preoccupied with fantasies about success, power, beauty, ideal love
- Feels unique or special
- Requires excessive admiration
- Entitlement expectations
- Interpersonally exploitative
- Lacks empathy
- Envious
- Arrogant/haughty

Other narcissistic traits**:
- Self-absorbed
- Self-admiring
- Perfectionist-compulsive
- Hypercompetitive
- Assertive
- Leadership
- Authoritative

---

*Adapted from Allnutt, S. and Links, P.S. Diagnosing specific personality disorders and the optimal criteria. In Clinical Assessment and Management of Severe Personality Disorders, ed. P.S. Links, Washington, DC: American Psychiatric Press, 1996, p. 36.

**Adapted from Watson, Paul J.; Morris, Ronald J.; and Miller, Liv. Narcissism and the self as continuum: correlations with assertiveness and hypercompetitiveness. Imagination, Cognition and Personality. 17(3):249–259, 1997–98; and Watson, Paul J.; Varnell, Sherri P.; and Morris, Ronald J. Self-reported narcissism and perfectionism: an ego-psychological perspective and the continuum hypothesis. Imagination, Cognition and Personality. 19(1):59–69, 2000.

Apropos of Watson's findings, it can be said that the healthy narcissist is able to experience a wide range of feelings deeply and demonstrate the ability to: accept recognition and awards when they are deserved, rather than regard them as to-the-manor born entitlements; disagree with an ideological adversary but not entertain a hatred toward him because of that disagreement; take reasonable pride in his accomplishments and objects of value but not feel animosity toward those who do not share that regard; feel a sting to his self-esteem when failure occurs, but be able to allocate responsibility for that failure objectively and emotionally recover from it; and feel reasonably comfortable in close relationships but not harbor dreadful anxieties about becoming engulfed or abandoned by them. Importantly, healthy narcissists will have the ability to soothe and recover from their painful feelings and not wallow in them to the extent that they become morose, bitter, or enraged.[8] The more advanced one's unhealthy narcissism is, however, the less he or she will be able to manage these kinds of emotional challenges.

The Pathological Narcissist

In speculating about the origins of the unhealthy narcissist, psychiatrist Michael Stone pointed out that:

> Narcissistic traits can develop, curiously, when there are deviations from ideal rearing on either side: pampering or neglecting; expecting too much or too little. Excessive praise of a child ... can give rise to ... feelings of superiority, of being destined for greatness ... But compensatory feelings of a similar kind can arise where there has been parental indifference and neglect, for in this situation a child may develop an exaggerated desire for "greatness" by way of shoring up a sense of self-worth in the absence of the ordinary parental praise. Whereas the overly praised child may regard himself as better than he really is, the neglected child may present a dual picture: an outward sense of (compensatory) specialness covering an inward sense of worthlessness.[9, p. 401]

Either the overindulgent or the emotionally distant parent fails to accomplish what the great British analyst Donald Winnicott claimed the "good-enough" parent does: to facilitate the child's development of a reliable network of feelings, attitudes, and beliefs about himself and the world that are regulated by a healthy sense of self, an appreciation of the independent existence of others, and appropriate feelings and beliefs about entitlements, responsibilities, and obligations.[10]

Psychiatrists have theorized that healthy psychological development consists, among other things, of the child's healthy development of both "mirroring" and "idealizing" transferences.[11] Mirroring transferences occur when the child understands and feels elated that the other—typically and most importantly his parent—is acknowledging and positively affirming his being. The mythical Narcissus experienced such a transference when he thought the reflection in the pond was adoring him—when it was, of course, only mirroring back to him the gaze and facial gestures that Narcissus was making in reaction to it. Children anticipate such transferences when they scream to their parents, "Mommy! Daddy! Watch me! Watch me!" Idealizing transferences occur when the individual understands an object—be it a person or experience like the practice of medicine—as sweeping, magnificent, and awesome and then proceeds to identify with it, saying, in effect, "*That* is what I want to be, what I want to devote myself to because it is so wonderful." Just so, Narcissus's idealizing perception of the intoxicatingly beautiful image in the pond witnessed his trying to embrace it and merge his being with it. (See Appendix 2.)

Unhealthy narcissists have a pathological need for such transferences. They desperately search out "perfect" objects or relationships that resonate with their feelings of specialness or superiority, and they relish praise and admiration from others because they are in constant need of self-affirmation. An unfortunate result of all this is that narcissists typically have great trouble forming authentically loving relationships. The pathological narcissist will spend his or her life depending on others to do what the parents did not, that is, affirm his or her lovability, value, and adequacy. Cultivating a self-structure of power, grandiosity, and perfection *as a defense against anxious feelings of unlovability and inadequacy*, the unhealthy narcissist develops relationships with others only insofar as they are useful in shoring up the narcissist's disrupted sense of self-esteem.[12]

As their primary psychological defense, narcissists develop a pathologically one-sided understanding of themselves as grandiose and marvelous and are constantly projecting this hopelessly idealized self-representation into their "object-representations," that is, their understanding of others in terms of how those others reflect, resonate, and confirm the narcissist's idealized self-understanding. The narcissist cannot love people authentically because he does not love himself authentically. Because he loves an idealized and exaggerated representation of himself and because he sees others only as they are in relation to this false, idealized self, the narcissist initially is inclined to project and love a fantasized representation of others who interest or attract him. When those others eventually fail to perfectly mirror the narcissist's self-idealization or when they assert their independence—that is, their being-for-themselves rather than their being just an extension of the narcissist's ego—the narcissist reacts with anger and dismissiveness.[13]

It is not a surprise that narcissists are notorious for their inability to tolerate painful truths about themselves as well as for the ease with which they become disaffected, disinterested, or enraged when the world does not accommodate their demands.[14] The unhealthy narcissist's entitlement fantasies are emanations of the grandiose self-structure that narcissists have developed as a defense against their insecurities. Whenever those insecurities are triggered by a *challenge* to their feelings of specialness or omnipotence, narcissists typically exhibit withdrawal, bewilderment, arrogance, or rage.[15]

The Narcissist as Special

A prominent psychological observation about narcissists is that many of them display a special talent or ability from early on.[16] As emotionally insecure but often gifted children, they quickly learn that they can parlay that ability or talent into being rewarded by the love and attention they crave. Identifying and then cultivating that special talent or skill, the budding narcissist *becomes* the beauty queen, the athlete, the scholar, the artist, the actor. Harboring either serious confusion or emotional doubts about their lovability, unhealthy narcissists—especially of the high-achieving ilk we will explore in this book—learn how to quell doubts about their value and preciousness through *outstanding* achievements (or what they hope will be understood as outstanding). Not surprisingly, parents of such children will often encourage the child's self-formation around this special, much admired trait since the child's accomplishments, and the public visibility those accomplishments attract, feed the parents' own need for narcissistic supplies.[17]

Consequently, the moment that marks both the boon and bane of the existence of unhealthy narcissists is when they begin *to derive intense satisfaction* in how their talents, skills, and beauty, enable them to manage their emotional vulnerabilities and affirm their grandiose self-image.[18] Unhealthy narcissists discover how their specialness or skills soothe their psychic fragility by attracting the respect and admiration of others; yet they are often suspicious about the authenticity of those very affections. They suspect that those affections are not inspired by who they really are but rather by some aspect of their self that was cultivated precisely for the purpose of attracting notice and glory. Yet, because that very talent or skill has proved itself a reliable vehicle for coping with the way life's disappointments challenge their sense of adequacy and value, the narcissistically attractive trait becomes the defining characteristic of their identity. If their narcissism progresses into serious pathology, they will exhibit certain feelings, beliefs, attitudes, and behaviors that typically include:

- A subjectively based insistence, originating from the narcissist's disrupted emotional core of self-doubt and insecurity, to act in accord with what his or her ideal self-image dictates
- An intensely defensive reaction toward anything that threatens the narcissist's ideal self-image
- A gradual loss of feeling for others, as the narcissist devotes more and more energy to merging with his or her ideal self
- An inordinate investment of energy and attention to merge with one's idealized self that causes other relationships to suffer
- A sometimes near-manic craving for success and achievement that will often witness the exploitation of others to attain that end
- A disowning of the real self, that is, the one who is flawed and imperfect.[19]

Always searching for that perfect love, many unhealthy narcissists are fooled into thinking that personal achievement or success is its means of acquisition. Furthermore, because the narcissist's ideal self embodies his or her self-adulatory fantasy, he or she denies or projects unappealing, unattractive, or pedestrian aspects of his or her actual self. This results in the narcissist's self-monitoring functions—which normally regulate one's self-understandings of responsibility and accountability—to become warped because the narcissist's self-idealization will not allow self-blame. Rather, he or she projects these negative representations onto others and hence regards them as inferior and lowly if they even hint at challenging the narcissist's self-esteem.[20]

Preview of What Is to Come. As a way of anticipating how all of this might apply to healthcare professionals, especially physicians, I will end this section by recalling a detail from one of the most memorable public lectures I ever attended. It was delivered by physician Eric Hedberg who described, in horrific detail, the onset of his drug dependency and his eventual, ongoing recovery. In the midst of the lecture, he described how physicians are encouraged to buy into what he called medicine's "12 Step Program," which consists of the following axioms:

WE:

1. Learned that we could handle everything, that we had total control
2. Came to believe there was no higher power than Medical Knowledge, that we ARE what we DO
3. Made a decision to turn our lives and our wills over to Medicine, resisting all need for self care
4. Made a searching and thorough inventory of Medical knowledge, committing it all to memory
5. Recognized that our discomforts are the faults of other people, places, and things and admitted no personal weaknesses
6. Denied our own negative feelings, doubts and misgivings
7. Never let our mistakes, fears, or feelings of inadequacy show and made preemptive strikes whenever possible
8. Made a list of all people, places, and things that upset us
9. Refused to resolve these tensions
10. Continued to act as if we were fine
11. Refused to accept new ideas, seeking only to live life on OUR TERMS
12. Rigidly cling to our original attitudes and ideas, recommending them to all aspiring Medical Professionals[21]

To the extent that these characterizations describe a minority but still goodly number of physicians, they stand as rather extraordinary corroborations of the narcissistic models that have been examined. Consider how item #1 is an unadulterated omnipotence fantasy, while item #2 implies an idealizing transference (i.e., "I shall be as great and powerful as medical knowledge itself."). Item #3 is a proud declaration of stoicism, but it suggests how the narcissist's overwhelming devotedness to his or her goals wreaks havoc with other aspects of his or her life. Item #4 smacks of both masochism and an omniscience fantasy, and items 5 and 6 are explicit examples of the narcissist who represses or splits off and then projects his or her own painful psychic materials onto others. Items #7 and #10 are frank admissions of the physician's need to protect and maintain the grandiose self, while item 8 expresses the narcissist's smoldering rage at all those who dare to challenge his special place in the universe. Items #9, #11, and #12 show how narcissistic physicians cannot give up the image they see reflected in Narcissus's pond.

Although this caricature admits the reality of highly unproductive, especially angry, and masochistic feelings, it ends by exalting and recommending its wisdom to all. It offers a model that presumably enables its adherents to keep from "falling apart," but with a modus vivendi that invites frustration and unhappiness.[22]

This characterization most certainly applies only to a small number of physicians, who might be considered arch medical narcissists. In the pages that follow, however, a more common, milder version of this kind of narcissist will be offered. Still in the minority of health professionals but commonly seen is the healthcare professional who is notable for his or her stubbornly unempathic behaviors. This is an individual who typically:

- Maintains a professional distance or guardedness with patients that largely precludes empathically reacting to their demonstrations of grief or suffering
- Insists on appearing utterly competent always (i.e., never admits weakness or fallibility)
- Understands and grounds that competence in scientific method and vocabulary
- Never admits ignorance or hesitation
- Always directs and controls the conversation with patients
- Uses the power of his or her white coat to direct how the patient ought to behave and feel

The following draws on clinical observations and some research that acknowledges this person's presence in healthcare and explains how this kind of medical narcissism could have developed. This material will also inform an understanding of how such a person might react to the commission of a medical error. I will begin with a discussion of two seminal papers by psychiatrist Glen O. Gabbard.

The "Medical Narcissist"

In a paper that Gabbard co-authored with Roy Menninger in 1988, entitled "The Psychology of the Physician," the following passage decidedly recalls key elements of the narcissistic etiology that is described above:

> The adult personality of the physician results from a defensive style adopted in early childhood to deal with what is perceived as parental failure to provide adequate emotional nurturance. This defensive style colors all subsequent relationships with patients, colleagues, and spouses … This is not to say that the parents of future physicians really were emotionally distant: the important point is that the physician sees them that way. Future physicians possibly require more parental encouragement and reassurance than the ordinary child if they are to feel loved and valued.[23, pp. 24–25]

The authors depict the physician going through life acting out his or her longings for mirroring transferences:

> The need to control others is also an important component of the doctor's personality. This involves … a wish to control the sources of love and support in the environment. Unconsciously, physicians expect that their

dedicated, selfless care will make others so grateful that they will respond with emotional support. The child felt essentially unloved; the adult feels a need to make heroic efforts to prove his or her value and receive the longed-for admiration.[24, p. 25]

Gabbard and Menninger sound the very common psychiatric observation that our behaviors, especially as they reflect important and ongoing life decisions and choices, are often born from and are defensive reactions toward experiences that cause us intense anxiety.[25] They speculate that the physician's narcissism proceeds from intense feelings of helplessness and vulnerability, such that the future physician strives for perfection and "wish(es) to live in the shadow of another person who is viewed as perfect. Perfectionism is so common in physicians that such prior feelings of helplessness and vulnerability must be common motivators in the choice of a medical career."[26, p. 27]

Well, these are remarkable claims. And a signal problem with them is that they are based on very little methodologically controlled data. For example, Gabbard's primary empirical support for thinking that children who become doctors suffer from a kind of impaired self-esteem is from a 1972 paper that reported the results of a 30-year study using questionnaire and interview data of 47 physicians.[27] By today's standards, this is a small sample size indeed while I'm not aware of any additional methodologically rigorous research that might confirm those findings.

Nevertheless, in a 2002 paper that describes the American Board of Internal Medicine's recent efforts to graduate humanistic (i.e., non-narcissistic) physicians, psychiatrist Donald Misch remarked on the methodological difficulty in just "defining and operationalizing humanism and its components such as compassion, empathy, caring integrity and respect."[28, p. 490] The absence of widely shared definitions of these terms as well as agreement on whether to study their expressions behaviorally, attitudinally, or cognitively also complicates any research on the psychological attributes of health professionals that aims at precision and exactness.

On the other hand, if the American Board of Internal Medicine is correct in noting that the "direct observation of physician behaviors is probably the most reliable, valid, and useful means of assessing physicians' professionalism and humanism,"[29, p. 490] then one can point to at least 15 years worth of qualitative research, observation, and anecdote that offer highly coherent reflections and respectable explanations for what we occasionally see as narcissistically based failures to accommodate the aspirations of humanistic medical care. Gabbard notes in another paper how the empirical findings he used to justify his claims on the narcissistic development of physicians are corroborated time and time again by clinical observation.[30] Additionally, one can point to the American Board of Internal Medicine's explicit concern about containing certain professional traits—especially arrogance, greed, misrepresentation, and lack of conscientiousness—that are decidedly narcissistic manifestations.[31, p. 529]

Consequently, I am going to proceed with some confidence (or perhaps, audacity) as well as with additional observations, data, and theoretical musings that the narcissistic portraits and characterizations that appear below are not unfamiliar among healthcare professionals and that they will be easily recognized by this book's readers; that they have considerable relevance for healthcare education; and that they have immense bearing on the degree to which healthcare relationships will or will not be therapeutic. While we should recognize that "pure" personality types such as the pathological and medical narcissistic types that are discussed in this chapter do not exist anywhere, the characterizations that appear below should resonate with many readers, along with the fact that they are at least somewhat supported by observational research that will be cited accordingly.

Narcissistic Vulnerability

As noted above but bears repeating, while certain health professionals may indeed manifest a pathological narcissism, the medical narcissist is typically of a different ilk. In fact, it is wrong to think that real-life narcissists embody a unitary or pure type of personality at all. As Paul Watson and his colleagues have shown repeatedly, the individual narcissist displays a cluster of positive and negative traits that place him or her at some point on a rather rough continuum that extends from marked maladjustment to robust emotional health.[32] Furthermore, if we refer to Figure 1, we can appreciate how the *magnitude* of any one of these traits in a person's narcissistic mix will differentiate narcissists from one another. The individual who strongly exhibits all the narcissistic traits included in the *Diagnostic and Statistical Manual of Mental Disorders* would resemble a modern-day Satan. Another kind of narcissist, however, might be very self-absorbed with marked feelings of specialness, entitlement, and hatred toward those who challenge him, but not be interpersonally exploitative or particularly lacking in empathy. Still another kind of narcissist, who decidedly verges toward a healthy narcissistic formation, might be one who displays marked assertiveness; leadership traits; always sounds authoritative and sometimes even haughty, but who also exhibits great empathy and caring; would not think to exploit others; and who consistently exhibits emotional maturity in absorbing his defeats and his victories.

What needs to be clear for now is that while grandiosity, poor self-esteem, excessive demand for admiration, and emotional exploitativeness might be the hallmarks of the "classic" pathological narcissist, emotional guardedness, lack of empathy, and controlling behaviors are the classic interpersonal characteristics of the medical narcissist. Most important, whereas the pathological narcissist sees the world as an extension of himself, the medical narcissist understands *medicine* as a primary conveyance for affirming his worth to the world. Consequently, when the medical narcissist encounters a clinical situation wherein he or she cannot make that proof—such as with end-of-life cases where treatment appears futile or, much worse, in cases of harm-causing medical error—the medical narcissist assumes the psychological armor of emotional distancing, often bordering on arrogance, as a way to cope with the challenge. Thus, in describing the dying of her significant other, British physician J. S. Maxmin captures the way health professionals use narcissistic-like defenses to ward off their anxieties over feeling inadequate:

> Nobody ever discussed his deterioration or prognosis. Diagnosis was all …
> I wonder whether the medical arrogance that I perceived was merely a
> mechanism to distance the doctors from our pain or from their sense of fail-
> ure. Was it an act of self-preservation? I can remember feeling ashamed that
> I was a doctor. It was what I perceived as a lack of compassion that was so
> shocking. The doctors seemed to be insulating themselves from their
> patient's suffering and in the absence of a cure, seemed to feel that they
> could offer nothing.[33, p. 684]

This is a superb description of the utility of a narcissistic trait, that is, emotional distancing, to serve as a psychological shield. Because these physicians could not call on
the one thing that enabled them to feel adequate or competent, namely their clinical
acumen and skill so as to effect a cure, their discomfort triggered self-protective intel-
lectualizations of what was happening that played out as arrogance.

    Yet, one of Maxmin's speculations bears repeating: It is quite possible that these
physicians' seemingly arrogant behaviors did not protect a pathologically disrupted or
fragile sense of self. Rather, their arrogance was "merely a mechanism to distance the
doctors from our pain or from their sense of failure." The mildest form of medical narcissism, then, is expressed by a cluster of interpersonal behaviors whose primary objective is to enable the professional to get through emotionally trying experiences. On the
other hand, there certainly are health professionals whose sense of self is so fragile that
when their need for narcissistic supplies is disappointed, they react in a markedly imma-
ture and nontherapeutic way. Indeed, when this more emotionally insecure medical narcissist encounters a particular kind of patient who he suspects at the outset will not
accommodate his expectation of narcissistic supplies, he or she might reject the patient
outright. An example of this is the account of a third-year medical student who observed
the following exchange between a surgeon and a prospective patient:

> Mrs. M was an extremely obese woman who appeared to have spent the last
> few days sleeping on the street—she was poorly dressed and extremely mal-
> odorous. She greeted us with hostility, telling us how much she hated and
> distrusted surgeons, and that she was merely seeing us out of courtesy to her
> internist, whom she very much respected. Lacking any patience, Dr. R.
> replied that if she felt this way then there was nothing he could offer. He
> pointed out that he believed she had an easily resectable tumor, but if it was
> not treated she might very well die from it. He carefully explained the pro-
> cedure, its risks and the possible complications. Mrs. M. reacted to his
> bluntness with anger and refused the operation. She got off the table and
> angrily left the room.
>
>   Dr. R was clearly frustrated by this interaction and reacted with some less
> than flattering remarks about Mrs. M's personality. I was also quite upset by
> this encounter. Here was a woman who had a potentially curable tumor
> walking away from help. My impression was that she had probably experi-
> enced a great deal of pain at the hands of physicians in the past and was not

willing to allow them to hurt her again. I felt that Dr. R in letting her leave the room had failed in his job in the most flagrant manner. Had he been more patient, more understanding of her fears, he might have been able to win her trust. I also felt that Dr. R did not like the patient and he implied that she was the type of person he did not like on his service.[34, p. 1130]

In this case, the surgeon makes no attempt to understand why the patient is oppositional, nor does he summon any energy to persuade her to consider the therapeutic possibility of a surgical cure. The medical student, who embodies a caring demeanor very typical of third-year students, is greatly upset by what he sees and by Dr. R's noting that the patient was the type he did not like on his service. It seems fair to speculate that Dr. R reacted to the patient in the cool and professionally distant way he did because this patient disappointed Dr. R's need for respect. Probably, too, she was so socio-culturally different from Dr. R that he could feel no resonance with her situation—another narcissistically based inability—that might otherwise trigger some sort of empathic concern for her welfare. Consequently, he felt that he was dispatching his professional responsibility by simply describing the operation and its risks and benefits. Perhaps, too, he did so in a tone of voice and in a matter-of-fact way that implied his disinterest in her disease and dislike of her as a human being. His narcissism, which largely consisted of a need to feel respected that this patient was clearly not accommodating, rendered him unable to summon any advocacy for her, resulting in his abandonment of this patient to her disease.

This story recalls Hedberg's item #11 in which certain, less well-adjusted medical narcissists will only want to proceed in caring for patients if the psychological dimensions of the treatment program accord with the narcissist's needs. Had the above patient been appropriately deferential or submissive, it would seem fair to anticipate that the surgeon would have carefully deployed his skills and summoned whatever energy was necessary to dispatch the surgery appropriately if not superbly. Important to note, the probability of this surgeon's acting beneficently as long as his narcissistic needs were accommodated serves to differentiate the medical narcissist from his or her more pathological counterpart: Deeply pathological narcissists only use people and have no real feelings for them. They exploit others and see them as vehicles for narcissistic self-aggrandizement. Medical narcissists, whatever the degree of their pathology, virtually cannot help but internalize and integrate a more healthy and wholesome view of others. For the medical narcissist to realize his goals of self-respect, admiration, and control, the patient's compliance and positive clinical outcome are crucial. Because health professionals must be somewhat appreciative of their patient's beliefs and psychological affects, and must at least recognize these phenomena *as belonging to the patient,* the medical narcissist is much more likely to maintain a degree of authentic regard for the other—or be able to implement more healthy object relations—than does the pathological narcissist. Whereas the stereotypical pathological narcissist has no feelings for others but only uses them as narcissistic supplies, only the most pathological or advanced medical narcissist will be entirely without a feeling capacity for others. Indeed, it is hard to imagine how such a person could graduate from medical or nursing school. On the other hand, what distinguishes the run-of-the-mill medical narcissist from other health professionals who permit themselves to feel empathy for their patients is that the medical narcissist is much more intent on protecting his authority and control from the external threat of a narcissistically injurious experience, such as occurred in the surgical scenario above.

Narcissistically based vulnerabilities are ubiquitous, however, and one need hardly be a card-carrying narcissist to feel the occasional need to call upon his or her defenses when a psychologically challenging situation assaults his or her sense of adequacy, ability, or control. Consider how the following might describe three levels of narcissistically based reactions to emotionally challenging patient encounters that any health professional might demonstrate:

- A first-level narcissistic response that is primarily triggered by anxiety. An example is when a patient asks a nurse or physician something like, "No one is talking to me. Am I dying?" To the extent this situation arouses anxiety in the professional, especially by way of inviting an emotionally uncomfortable conversation that might make the health professional feel helpless, the professional might resort to some variety of evasion by which he or she will attempt to ignore or dismiss the patient's remark (e.g., "Hey, we're all dying."), or have the patient refocus attention on something else (e.g., "Oh, don't ask such questions. Let's concentrate on your treatment this afternoon."), or cajole or use humor (e.g., "I don't think it's time to sell the furniture yet, Mr. Jones."), or be overly reassuring, distract the patient, or distort or reinterpret the patient's concern.

- A second-level response that is primarily triggered by anger. Here, the professional experiences his or her adequacy at much greater threat and responds more forcefully. An example is the patient who accuses his or her treating physician or nurses of gross incompetence. Typical level-two defensive responses are withdrawal from the patient, or lecturing, sermonizing, arguing, threatening, or blaming—all geared toward the professional's need to assert his or her rightful authority so as to regain sufficient control of the situation and repair his or her damaged self-esteem.

- A third-level response as triggered by feelings of extreme anger and hatred. Patients who are sociopathic, extremely abrasive, obstreperous, or utterly noncompliant might elicit the health professional's unmitigated rage. Here, the professional whose composure and self-esteem have been completely overturned may be tempted to hurt back, such as the surgeon did by acting toward the disrespectful patient with a resectable tumor in a way that was unconsciously or consciously designed to result in her refusing care and perhaps succumbing to an otherwise curable disease. I will never forget a lecture delivered by a distinguished psychiatrist to a group of medical students. At one point he said to them, "You will meet many patients in your careers whom you will want to harm. Try not to hurt them too much."

As implied in the second item of Eric Hedberg's Medicine's 12 Step Program, the medical narcissist's fulfillment requires his or her deploying treatment as a means of securing self-affirmation. All medical narcissists, whatever their degree of emotional adjustment, demonstrate this phenomenon, and this defense mechanism will be prominent in the case study of the next chapter. When they are deprived of this narcissistic "fix," they are at a loss since medical narcissists suppress that part of their selves that can be supportive and empathic.

Making the Medical Narcissist

Childhood Antecedents and Familial Enablings

Anecdotal observation suggests that about 10 to 40 percent of students in any medical school class have at least one parent who is a physician, while about 30 to 50 percent have at least one parent who is a healthcare professional.[35] We have already seen Gabbard's and Menninger's speculation that, as children, physicians experienced failures of parental empathy such that they developed a dedicated work ethic aimed at sterling achievement in order to secure the admiration and respect they felt was withheld from them. It is extremely difficult to accept that claim as categorically true although it may indeed be true for more physicians than we think (as well as for many other, hard-driving professionals).

Yet, Martin Leichtman, who has done therapeutic work with physician families, noted that, "many of the doctors in our groups were themselves children of doctors," and paid the price that so many children of physician or professional fathers do: be without his physical or emotional presence for much of the time as well as identify with a fierce work ethic.[36]

Leichtman found that male doctors typically define themselves as physicians first and spouses and parents second. In "turning their lives and wills over to medicine" as Hedberg's item #3 recalls, certain physicians largely leave the upbringing of the children to their wives. Now, while Leichtman's 20-year-old gender stereotype of physician fathers who have wives as homemakers is robustly changing today, if physicians practicing today had a physician parent, that parent was most likely the father. Furthermore, and what has become virtually a clichéd observation in the literature on narcissism, narcissists overwhelmingly tend to be male and either an only child or a first-born.[37] Leichtman opined that if the child is a first-born, he or she may have to become self-reliant for love and affection because other children will be on the way. The child may feel he cannot depend on unconditional affection from a father who is rarely present or a mother who may be overwhelmed with running a household and who, indeed, may resent the way she has become a full-time, virtually single parent. Furthermore, to the extent that the mother has given up a career or her achievement hopes to raise her children, those children can become substitute vehicles of success if they assume the behaviors and attitudes that she approves. She may therefore become extremely demanding that her children rapidly mature, and she might use her own affection as a tool toward that end. Leichtman speculates that:

> When a woman has sacrificed her own career and goals, the child is "special," becoming the carrier of her own aspirations and the proof of her creativity as a parent. A child who seems mature and sensitive from an early age can also become a source of comfort and companionship to the mother, filling a vacuum left by her husband. Such "specialness" has a price. True autonomy, the freedom to pursue one's own life, is reduced. Meanwhile the child is pressured to ignore and deny regressive or dependent wishes while constantly striving to succeed. The child's character structure may then begin to resemble the father's.[38, p. 110]

Of course, it is a fact that many students who enter medical school commonly have high-achieving parents and that these very students usually display immense, sometimes astonishing academic prowess. Moreover, it may well be that the (especially male) child whose professional father is frequently absent or, even when present, seems emotionally unavailable, either comes to identify with the father's behavior by way of developing self-reliance and independence, or experiences intense anger at both the mother and father's emotional distance or manipulation.[39]

Later development. But even if psychological factors that can foster narcissistic inclinations are absent in the individual's childhood and the child develops a healthy sense of self, as an adult health professional, especially as a male physician with a family, he might experience a perfect environment for unhealthy narcissistic inclinations to blossom. Most male physicians marry while they are in training, and their wives quickly learn that their husbands will frequently be absent. Anecdotes abound at how frustrating it can be for wives to feel abandoned, but how they also feel unable to object when the duty of medicine calls. Family members can easily come to feel that their need for the love and support of their physician father and physician husband must take second place to others whose very lives may depend on the physician's presence. As such, Leichtman contends that a familial structure can evolve that resigns itself to the absent father-physician, such that the mother and children may enter into an emotional collusion:

> Physicians have outside sources of satisfaction; their wives often do not. As a result, mothers and children may band together to exclude fathers from family life; or children, sensitive to their parents' unhappiness, may be placed in or adopt roles designed to meet their parents' needs and balance the family system.[40, p. 112]

Again, the child finds him- or herself manipulated to soothe familial tensions and may very well adopt the parents' coping patterns, especially as they bear on emotional separateness, withdrawal, and self-reliance. Leichtman gives a sad example from his clinical work that illustrates how a physician parent with an advanced narcissism glowed when his emotionally troubled son acknowledged the nobility of his father's work:

> An example is Kurt, a serious, rather depressed 16 years-old [sic] who accompanied his parents to one of the workshops (for medical marriages and families) ... [Kurt's] father stood out in a group of 25 physicians because he flaunted his overriding commitment to medical values above all else. He actually embarrassed the others, who saw him as a caricature of the ideal physician ... Physicians and wives in this group spent much of the workshop trying to help the family, but Kurt's father seemed indifferent to what they said.
>
> The leaders of the group hoped that during the adolescent panel Kurt's father might finally listen. It was not to be. When Kurt spoke, he kept his eyes on his father and endorsed fully his father's values and style of life, while the father beamed with pleasure. Undoubtedly, Kurt feared his father's displeasure and desperately wanted his approval. But he probably also felt protective, sensing that the man's rigidity was accompanied by fragility and extreme vulnerability.[41, p. 116]

Medical Training, Protecting the Self, and the Cultivation of Omniscience and Omnipotence Fantasies

The Impressionable Student. What has just been discussed describes a familial dynamic that inclines the future medical narcissist toward a less well-adjusted self. Now consider how a relatively well-adjusted individual entering medical training might discover an environment that encourages the development of a perfectionist, even grandiose sense of self. If we look for explanations as to why many student-doctors begin their training with categorically empathic ideals only to graduate from their residency programs 8 to 12 years later jaded, cynical, and adverting to narcissistic behaviors and relational styles as psychological strategies by which to cope, one place to start is with the immensely anxiety-provoking environment of healthcare itself. As one medical anthropologist put it: "The world of a doctor ... has a peculiar code of heroics, self-denial, and stress—it's a culture of stress."[42, p. 26]

And not just for physicians. Patricia Benner is widely known for her qualitative research on the evolution of nursing expertise. Benner noted how beginner nurses often feel a dreadful lack of confidence in their knowledge and ability when her interviewees frequently alluded to the reliance they placed on formal standards of care, unit procedures, physician and nurses' orders, and patient records.[43] In the hundreds of interviews she did with nurses at various stages of their careers, Benner found that beginners particularly remarked that they rarely rejected or seriously doubted the authority of more experienced clinicians, and that they constantly observed the actions of more veteran staff to discern how to determine salience and what and when action is required.[44]

These nurses, however psychologically healthy they might otherwise be, do not as yet have enough confidence in their clinical intuitions for the entirely understandable reason that they have not had the requisite experience whereby such confidence becomes warranted.

Beginner nurses are also acutely aware that they are often acting at the outer edge of their ability, which considerably adds to their anxiety and their self-consciousness. Excessive self-consciousness is itself a kind of narcissistic phenomenon, although for most, it is a temporary moment in the evolution of the professional self. For example, when a beginner nurse who had just participated in her first cardiopulmonary resuscitation attempt was asked how she felt when it was over, she replied: "I felt relieved that I had made it through it and I had made the right decisions … I think the major thing was that I had survived it, so if it happens again, I'll know what to do."[45, p. 58]

While the nurse's use of "survived" is ironic, it nevertheless shows her acute self-consciousness. Benner notes that the beginner health professional wants desperately to feel kinship with her peers and so is often acutely sensitive to the cultural norms of her unit so that she can behave accordingly.

Just so with student physicians. In a frequently cited paper, Feudtner and Christakis noted:

> Even though students do begin medical school with core values, our experience has shown that they are hardly immutable—the fabric of their ethical beliefs can be unraveled, tattered, and even rewoven. It would seem to make more sense, then, to speak of an emerging "ethical self": a composite entity that encompasses not only individuals' evolving personal values but also the operational rules for handling ethical dilemmas that they adopt from their colleagues and institutions … Engulfed in these often bewildering surroundings, with their lofty expectations, students usually find security by becoming diligent members of the team.[46, p. 7]

What happens, then, when an impressionable, anxious, eager-to-please, developing professional self witnesses grossly unprofessional and unethical behavior toward patients? In a number of studies, medical students reported how they observed patients who were deceived and manipulated into taking medicines they did not want; patients who were sedated and then used for "practice" (e.g., having medical students do cervical examinations on an unconscious, nonconsenting patient); treatment notes written about patients who, in fact, were never seen; orders written and signed using the intern's name with the intern's full knowledge and approval; the omission of certain findings from the patient's chart because of further work-up that the finding would entail; and students who were instructed to conceal examination findings (e.g., cancer) from patients or, if the patient asks, to just lie.[47]

The unreflective, unquestioning student health professional who witnesses and then understands these practices as perfectly acceptable professional-patient interactions is learning how to be a narcissist: to take the power, authority, and centrality of the health professional role for granted and to dismiss the idea of patient dignity or patient rights as ideological nonsense. Howard Spiro, former Director of the Program for Humanities in Medicine at Yale, ruefully remarked, "Physicians are trained in narcissism" in that these kinds of training experiences can turn the concept of "patient-centered" rights and sensibilities into a canard.[48, p. 9]

The Patient as Enemy. On the other hand, sometimes patients simply appear to be the enemy. Probably every health provider can relate to the following story, told by a second-year resident:

> One night when I was really exhausted … this patient came in by ambulance with a heart attack. It was four in the morning, and I'd been up since eight the morning before, and up late working the night before that. They gave her streptokinase, a clot dissolver, in the ambulance to break up a clot in her coronary artery. This medicine can cause a person's heart to become very unstable. They can arrest and code multiple times. I remember being so tired and pissed off that I didn't know how to manage this patient. I wasn't getting any supervision, and I remember thinking, God, I wish this woman would just die. She kept coding, and it was like she was torturing me. I took it very personally. This was a horrible experience for me. I still feel guilty.[49, p. 113]

The contribution of these kinds of events to a nascent narcissism consists in how they present a schizoid message to physicians who are told they must be empathic, caring, and available, and yet are made to work indescribably grueling hours and tolerate emotional anguish that exists in no other profession. If the difficult-to-treat patient can sometimes represent the "enemy," then he or she presents a challenge to the physician's very survival. In such situations, it is easy to see how physicians will come to valorize their own welfare over the very individuals they are duty bound to care for. In a *New England Journal of Medicine* article, Timothy McCall similarly noted how a resident physician's protecting his or her self in these kinds of situations becomes a means of survival:

> House officers (i.e., residents) can be ruthless in preserving the precious hour or two of sleep they may be able to take while on call … Rather than replace a patient's intravenous line in the middle of the night, they routinely substitute intramuscular medications, ignoring the question of patient discomfort and the possibility of more erratic absorption of the drug.[50, p. 776]

Omnipotence Fantasies. The kinds of experiences described above encourage an attitude of self-centeredness that is understandably born from the physician's need to survive from day to day. Physicians still in residency training learn that they must protect themselves just to keep from being physically and emotionally destroyed. But these kinds of experiences can also encourage a related and even more compelling moment in the development of a physician's narcissistic self—that is, their encouraging omniscience and omnipotence *fantasies* by which the professional can cope with the emotionally turbulent and abusive world that medicine frequently is.

In his book, *Residents,* David Ewing Duncan describes how physicians just out of medical school as first-year interns or residents are suddenly given patient care responsibilities whose scope and magnitude far exceed their ability.[51] Although this phenomenon is a pedagogical mainstay of medical training, it is in itself an unwitting contributor to a narcissistic formation because it tokens a philosophy of training "so biased toward experience that educators and senior physicians are willing to take chances (i.e., with patients' welfare)."[52, p. 55] As physician Bertrand Bell, who chaired the 1987 New York state commission that first suggested significantly limiting resident work hours and increasing residents' supervision, said, "When people finish medical school, they can't take care of a cat. But they're expected to know everything in medicine on the first day they start as an intern. They are left as the front line to tend the patients, and they know next to nothing that's not in a book. This is madness."[53, p. 57]

It is hardly surprising that some of these individuals will evolve narcissistic fantasies of omnipotence just to cope with their discomfort of shouldering so much responsibility with so little preparation. Convincing oneself that he or she can handle any situation—indeed, that he or she is indestructible—turns what would normally be a flight of fancy into a literal belief and, as Gabbard recalls, "is a way of fending off a continuing sense of inadequacy."[54, p. 28] I recall a resident telling me that in her intern year, she had mononucleosis for six weeks before she had it diagnosed and treated because, "I thought everybody I was training with felt this way." Duncan tells the bizarre story of a second-year resident who contracted hepatitis:

> ...and hooked himself up to an I.V. pump attached to a portable pole. With antibiotics and fluids dripping into veins, he persisted in treating patients and performing his usual duties for two or three days, until his chief finally made him go home.[55, p. 107]

In any number of clinical scenarios, the professional's need to persuade himself of his competency so as to control his anxiety becomes paramount and can be readily accomplished by his replacing every shred of self-doubt with fantasies of omnipotence, blaming others when things go wrong, numbing himself to whatever emotional discomfort might be present and, as we have seen, cognitively distorting or reinterpreting a clinical event so as to be relieved of its psychical pain. Eric Marcus, a psychiatrist who studied the dreams of medical students and physicians, remarked about the "grandiose knowledge fantasies" of medical students as ways of protecting themselves from their terror of hurting or killing patients. Marcus describes these young, inexperienced physicians as oscillating among their omnipotence fantasies, their belief that they will master the entirety of clinical knowledge, and the "humiliating deflation" they experience in realizing that doing so is impossible.[56]

Note, too, that these fantasies occur in tandem with the way many resident physicians absorb perfectionistic standards from their attending supervisors. Duncan quoted one resident who said:

> [W]hen you reach a certain level of fatigue, the thing that keeps you going is not your concern for the patient. I hate to admit it. It's the knowledge that

someone senior to you has expectations of you, and, by God, you better not fail them.[57, p. 151]

The oppressive and sometimes sadistic physician-supervisor breeds what Glen Gabbard remarked is at the core of the physician's personality: compulsiveness. Driving oneself to take good care of patients so as to please one's supervisor suggests how the resident's "superego" development is shaped by the harshness and discipline of his or her senior physician. Important to note is that nascent compulsivity does not only develop for the patient's sake but, true to compensatory narcissistic form, is engineered by the supervisor-parental figure so as to be internalized by the student.

Deification Projections. This chapter would be remiss not to mention one more source of medical narcissism: what might be called "deification projections" from patients. Projection is a remarkably common phenomenon in healthcare that occurs when patients seek to "share" their feelings with those around them. Projection serves a twofold purpose of 1) enabling one individual—in this case, the health professional—to gain a glimpse into what the projector-patient is feeling, and 2) displacing the painful psychical content from the patient to the professional, and thus help the patient feel better.[58]

An instructional videotape I sometimes use with medical students begins with a medical student finishing a brief examination of a 60-year-old woman who is terminally ill. As he prepares to leave, the patient looks at him and feebly asks, "What do they teach you to say to dying old ladies like me?" Taken aback, he stares at her for a moment and then replies, "You've got breakfast on your nightgown. I see oatmeal and I see strawberry jam."[59] This exchange brilliantly captures the way patients want their health providers to comprehend what the patient is experiencing and feeling, but it also illustrates the way many professionals poorly—indeed, narcissistically—handle the projection. The patient wants the physician to imagine what it is like to be her, but he finds this unpleasant, and he cleverly diverts her attention to something else. Recall how in Mr. Thompson's insulin dosing error described in the previous chapter, the physician responded to his anger by admonishing him not to yell, when, in fact, Mr. Thompson had a perfect right to be upset. The physician could not tolerate his projection of negative emotional content and chided him for inappropriate behavior.

But it is hardly the case that all projections are painful. The physician who encounters a patient who literally deifies him may powerfully absorb that projection and come to internalize and integrate that feeling as part of his self-structure. Writing about arrogance among physicians, Allan Berger pointed to:

> …the tendency of the very ill and suffering patient to regress psychologically to a childlike emotional state in which the physician is unconsciously viewed as an omnipotent and omniscient parent who is sure to protect and save the suffering child … [T]his regression, with its accompanying tendency to idealize and deify the doctor and expect miracles, is directly proportional to the gravity of the illness, the patient's state of consciousness, and the drama of the occasion … The patient's longing for an omnipotent

physician/parent God to save him or her taps into the latent arrogance/ grandiosity/hubris of some physicians. In effect, the patient is unknowingly fostering the very physician attribute of arrogance that the patient, as well as society, decries.[60, pp. 146–147]

Indeed, one would think that such deification projections are so common that it is amazing that so many health professionals, indeed the majority in my experience, understand them for what they are and do not succumb to them. But to the individual with a proclivity toward unhealthy narcissism, these projections are narcissistic aphrodisiacs.

The above illustrates certain formative experiences of medical narcissists. In what follows, I want to describe in some detail three rather common personality characteristics of such individuals: their lack of empathy, their ideological rigidity, and their compulsiveness. Along the way, I will continue to discuss how individuals whose narcissism has taken on these forms differ from the classic pathological narcissist, but I want now to speculate on how the medical narcissist might respond to the commission of a medical error and manage or mismanage its disclosure to a harmed party.

Three Characteristics of Medical Narcissists and Their Applications to Medical Error

Emotional Disengagement

Because it constitutes the quintessence of self-centeredness, narcissism is the antithesis of the caring, patient-centered attitude. But if one of medical narcissism's functions is to protect one from the emotional abuse and feelings of inadequacy that are inevitable in caring for the sick, then narcissistic behaviors offer a certain amount of survival value. In the world of healthcare, as Dr. Maxmin learned, perhaps a predictable moment is an occasional encounter with an emotionally distant, self-centered, defensive, overly intellectualizing professional whose interpersonal style helps him or her survive the emotional turbulence of taking care of people who are sick and miserable.

Emotional disengagement is a hallmark characteristic of either pathological or medical narcissism. While a pathological narcissist's excessive self-preoccupation leaves him little psychical energy or interest in the feelings of others, it appears that many health professionals form a decided but misinformed belief early in their careers that emotional distancing and disengagement are important survival strategies. Patients and their significant others are constantly projecting their misery onto health professionals, which can trigger exactly the kinds of uncomfortable feelings that a health professional's narcissism is poised to fend off. The result of the latter's reactions becomes the health professional's "unempathic" persona that patients interpret for indifference or arrogance.

Empathy, which we will understand as the professional's attempt to imagine the patient's feelings and understanding of his situation, connotes the polar opposite of narcissism. Despite his fame as an exemplary physician and teacher, William Osler set the aspirations of empathy back a century with his most famous essay "Aequanimitas," in which he recommended that:

> [I]n the physician or surgeon no quality takes rank with imperturbability ... an inscrutable face may prove a fortune ... a certain measure of insensibility is not only an advantage, but a positive necessity ... [F]or the practitioner in his working-day work, a callousness which thinks only of the good to be effected, and goes ahead regardless of smaller considerations, is the preferable quality.[61, pp. 23 and 25]

Searching for a biological simile that expresses this demeanor, Osler hit upon "phlegm": "Imperturbability means ... immobility, impassiveness, or, to use an old and expressive word, *phlegm.*"[62, p. 24]

But psychiatrist Jodi Halpern recently and impressively argued that patients may be inclined to understand this Oslerian emotional detachment, which has nevertheless been reverentially passed down to generations of physicians, as indifference.[63] Osler's emphasis on "clinical objectivity" may robustly encourage a health professional's narcissism in that it provides a time-honored excuse for the emotional noninvolvement that characterizes the comprehension and treatment of disease in a purely materialist-reductionist way.[64]

Perhaps the most common way that health professionals effect emotional disengagement while simultaneously preserving their narcissistic personae of competence and adequacy is by becoming excessively focused on the treatment they are to deliver. These individuals find that being fixated on treatment (FOT) can serve as a shield or substitute for their lack of empathy toward the patient's emotional suffering and concern. Moreover, by endlessly honing and polishing their treatment skills, they often evolve a terrific, narcissistically based pride that can progress into an overweening, unbounded, and unrealistic confidence about their ability. In what follows, I will call these individuals FOTs.

Sadly and reminiscent of Maxmin's experience with the physicians treating her dying lover, the FOT learns not to relate primarily to human beings but rather to their diseases and especially to whatever intervention he or she is trained to deploy in diagnosis or treatment. The pathological content of the FOT's narcissism is a combination of fantasized omnipotence and a covert desire for adulation, which FOTs believe they can attain through mastering clinical interventions. While there is nothing wrong with a health professional who takes great pride in his or her skills, the FOT's insecurities and anxieties cause him to concentrate on his clinical prowess to such a degree that it overwhelms whatever interest or energy he might otherwise devote to the humanistic trappings of the patient encounter. Thus, the patient who says to the FOT, "My God, I never had back pain like that in my life. I actually began to cry. I thought I would be better off dead, and then I seriously thought that I was going to die," might hear in return, "Hmmm, did the pain radiate up your neck?"

Surgeons—who, after all, operate in a "theater"—are the literature's favorite, narcissistic FOTs. Stereotypically, they are preoccupied with technique; they oscillate between feelings of veneration and envy for their leaders and teachers; they are notorious for resisting empathic conversation with their patients; they are known to be extremely action-oriented and to disdain the kind of thoughtful approach to clinical situations typical of other specialists like internists or neurologists; they couch information to their patients in an augustly technical and largely incomprehensible vocabulary; they shrink from discussing emotionally unpleasant information with patients despite their swashbuckling personae; and not surprisingly, they are the most likely physician-specialty group to be sued, not because of technical incompetence but because of strident patient complaints about their poor relational skills.[65]

But the FOT need hardly be a surgeon. In her memoirs, Alma Mahler-Werfels gives a brief but exquisite description of a famous bacteriologist named Chantemesse, who was secured in the hope that he might be able to cure Alma's dying husband, the great conductor and composer, Gustav Mahler. She wrote that Chantemesse:

> . . .made a culture of Mahler's blood and appeared a few days later with a microscope, beaming. Had a miracle happened?
>
> The famous man adjusted his microscope. 'Look in here, Madame Mahler. Even I have never seen such marvelously developed streptococci. Look at these strands—like seaweed!'
>
> He wanted to explain further, but I left the room.[66, pp. 63-64]

Chantemesse compensated for his failure to be of value to the Mahlers by exulting in his discovery of the pathogen. His narcissism blinded him to the incongruity of his elation in the face of Alma's anguish over her husband's impending death. But self-absorbed professionals like Chantemesse are likely to be disinterested in their patient's feelings and are often poor listeners. Because they venerate and identify with what they do, which recalls Hedberg's axiom #2, they believe that the only worthwhile conversation with patients is to discuss its aspects and merits.[67]

When things go well, the therapy and, by extension, the therapist take the credit. Therapeutic success and the patient's gratitude are the FOT's reward. When things go poorly, FOTs will often blame extra-clinical factors. Stephen Macciocchi and Bradford Eaton, for example, surveyed 51 neurorehabilitation therapists selected from various disciplines (e.g., occupational therapy, physical therapy, speech therapy, and recreation therapy) and asked them to list factors that are responsible for poor versus favorable outcomes from brain injury or stroke.[68] Now, it is well known that the single factor that most influences outcome from these neurological insults is the severity of the individual's initial injury. Macciocchi and Eaton found, however, that if therapists were asked to list outcome factors, only 20 percent cited injury severity as among the first five outcome factors. On the other hand, when the therapists were provided with a written list of factors that could potentially affect outcome—that is, when they were cued with outcome variables and asked to select from the list—80 percent ranked injury severity as the most important factor. Equally interesting, though, is the researchers' finding that, "therapists also attributed positive outcomes in neurorehabilitation to their skill, treatment programs, and team process while attributing unsuccessful outcomes to factors outside the therapist's control." [69, p. 523]

If this exaggerated valorizing of clinical skills is in any way representative, it is not surprising that when the effectiveness of those very skills is challenged, certain health professionals will respond poorly. Patients who question the FOT's judgments, ask for second opinions, or inquire about alternative remedies can be extremely annoying to the FOT because such questions challenge what the professional is offering and, by extension, the professional him- or herself. Because such patients can trigger the very anxieties that the FOT's narcissism is meant to manage, these patients are labeled "difficult," and the professional's response to them is silence, argument, disdain, or sometimes a flat refusal to care for them.[70] Thus, the occurrence of a poor outcome that was unanticipated, or worse, was due to error is very likely to arouse whatever insecurities the FOT may have. The rather considerable body of literature that attests to the ways professionals react to such situations—resisting communications with patients, rationalizing what happened as depicted in the previous chapter, or looking for others to blame—illustrates the kind of relational damage their narcissistic formations can do.[71]

The Emotionally Disengaged Professional's Reaction to Medical Error

Persons who learned to be emotionally disengaged from their patient's experience are likely to respond to medical errors in a relationally clumsy fashion. While they might very well acknowledge an error when they see it, their management of its aftermath, especially per its communication to the patient, can be an empathic disaster. They will be especially hard-pressed to appreciate the impact of error disclosure from the standpoint of the patient's subjective experience (like the physician involved with Mr. Thompson and his insulin dosage error in the previous chapter). FOTs who are thoroughly traumatized by an error might be tempted to confabulate it as a "learning experience" and work hard to rationalize its concealment, or obfuscate or rationalize the error in the ways we examined previously. The FOT's anxiety over having to admit that the very thing which he or she venerates was at fault, namely his or her treatment acumen or skill, will provoke immense discomfort. Consequently, FOTs may be extremely disinclined from using words like "error" or "mistake" in their disclosure and would rather disclose in a manner that Thomas Gallagher and his colleagues found typical: in extremely parsimonious bits and pieces that resist admitting error except if the patient is relentless in asking probing questions.[72]

Ideological Rigidity

Some persons arrive at the beginning of their healthcare training with firm ideological values and attitudes. They are so deeply convinced of the truth of their beliefs about human responsibility, justice, and the like that they are reflexively dismissive of, or at least never persuaded by, others with contrasting beliefs. The rigidity and immense passion that characterize their convictions suggest deeply defensive reactions to the possibility that they might be wrong.[73]

Like all the narcissistic manifestations we have been examining, people with very rigid cultural and ideological beliefs have considerable difficulty reaching out to others because doing so not only requires them to exert imaginative insight into how another person understands the world, but it also requires a continuing commitment to that other person's values and experiences.[74] Performing either psychological activity is immensely difficult for anyone whose narcissism is fairly advanced.

Additionally, many U.S. health professionals, including otherwise healthy non-narcissistic personality types, have considerable difficulty sustaining an authentic respect and curiosity for cultural values that understand the meaning of health and the nature of healthcare differently from the Western, Newtonian, germ-theory perspective.[75] Western-trained health professionals are singularly steeped in a biophysiological account of disease and illness that comprehends diseases as molecular, cellular, and organic phenomena. But because patients do not experience their molecules but rather the various feelings and emotions that attach to their illnesses, the Western approach has a tendency to subtract the patient from the illness. If patients wonder why the health professional is not more interested in their personal experience of the illness, it is because many health professionals have not been taught about the importance of that subjective understanding and to be sensitive to the beliefs that sustain it.[76] Furthermore, it is quite likely that many health professionals associate their sense of professional adequacy with their mastery of a particular body of knowledge. The patient, therefore, who evinces little respect for that knowledge, such as the one who expresses great confidence in alternative and complementary medical approaches, can easily upset this kind of medical narcissist.

A related manifestation of this health professional's narcissism is his or her having great difficulty in relating to persons *unlike* him or her, such as was illustrated in the surgical case at the beginning of this chapter. These narcissists can be found in any professional discipline. In her collaborative study of nurses with Patricia Benner, Jane Rubin remarked about certain nurses who:

> ...insofar as they do acknowledge a realm of individual, subjective, meaning ... assume that their patients will find the same meaning in the situation that they, the nurses, imagine they would find if they were in a similar situation. Indeed, these nurses seem to be able to establish a relationship with a patient only to the extent that they can imagine that that patient's experience is the same as their own ... These nurses never come to experience their patients as individuals.[77, p. 176–177]

Given Rubin's description, these individuals certainly sound like or verge toward an unhealthy narcissism, and yet we should consider the possibility that, for all their ideological self-centeredness and posturing, many of them may be relatively well adjusted. If there is any determinative factor that tips the balance of psychological health one way or another among these persons, it would be in the way they can sustain the passion of their convictions without compromising the therapeutic relationship. In other words, to the extent that Rubin's nurses, when confronted with situations that challenge their valuative elitism or self-centeredness, defensively react by lecturing, sermonizing, rationalizing, blaming, or simply dismissing the other's beliefs, they verge toward the pathological pole of Paul Watson's narcissistic continuum discussed earlier. To the extent that they let their ideological disagreements with the patient be known but simultaneously assure the patient that such disagreement will not interfere with his or her care, they verge toward the better-adjusted end. With the caveat that even the haughty health professional can sustain a therapeutic professional-patient relationship, I will refer to these individuals as haughty, ideologically rigid professionals or HIRPs.

How HIRPs Respond to Error

If a HIRP is also compulsive or perfectionistic, he or she is likely to be devastated by serious, harm-causing error. Rigidity combined with perfectionistic expectations of oneself has the makings for major psychological trauma in the face of evidence of one's incompetence. On the other hand, if this individual only assumes a posture of ideological and cultural inflexibility for the psychological comfort it affords and is without the perfectionistic aspirations of many other medical narcissists, there is little way of predicting how HIRPs will respond to error. While the HIRP may not be particularly empathic, that hardly implies that he or she will lose sight of his or her moral obligation, and conceal or obfuscate the error. The HIRP might be devastated by the error because, for example, the error is acutely embarrassing evidence of the HIRP's failure to live up to his or her self-image.

Individuals who harbor axiomatic and rigid understandings of relational responsibilities seem often to favor a contractual model for comprehending the patient-professional relationship. A contractual model whose terms define who is responsible for what relieves the HIRP of the messy job of empathically understanding the patient's experience since the HIRP often becomes uncomfortable trying to understand why a dispute exists, what values are at stake, or how a valuative negotiation might be realized in the midst of conflict. As James Childress pointed out, a contractual model "neglect(s) the virtues of benevolence, care, and compassion that are stressed in other models such as paternalism and friendship."[78, p. 47] Of course, the HIRP will likely insist that the terms of the contract be his or her own, not the patient's. Indeed, it is not beyond the realm of possibility that a key party that HIRPs might be tempted to target in allocating responsibility for error is their patient—as health professionals are often used to beleaguering patients about the latters' responsibility for their conditions or clinical progress. It is hardly a significant stretch for certain unhealthily narcissistic HIRPs to extend whatever patient-blaming attitudes they have already developed in caring for "difficult" patients to instances of medical error, if they sense even the dimmest possibility that the harm-causing error might not be entirely their fault. So that had the patient "not been so obese, or noncompliant, or been better educated, or better supported, or had better insurance," the error would not have occurred or, more likely, its resulting harm would not have been so grave.

Amazingly, in 1896, Freud was himself guilty of just such a transfer of blame to a patient, named Emma Eckstein, who was harmed by error.[79] Since 1887, Freud had corresponded and then collaborated with an ear, nose, and throat specialist named Wilhelm Fliess, who practiced in Berlin. Whereas Freud's ideas on the sexual origins of the neuroses were evolving during those years, Fliess advanced the notion of the sexual importance of the nose and published in 1897 *The Nose and the Female Sex Organs*. In that book, Fliess claimed that a complex relationship existed among the nose, the female sex organs, and the menstrual process and that:

> The pathology of menstruation finds its reflection in birth: the same mechanisms and the same conditions that hold true for nasal dysmenorrhea also control the pains of contraction.[80, p. 19]

In fact, Fliess believed that an abortion could be stimulated through a woman's nose. Emma Eckstein suffered from menstrual and stomach discomforts, and Freud asked Fliess to do nasal surgery on Eckstein in the belief that operating on her nose would favorably affect her dysmenorrhea.

So, Fliess traveled from Berlin to Vienna, performed the operation on Emma, which appeared to be a success, and returned to Berlin. Two weeks later, however, Emma began to hemorrhage from her nose, and in the days that followed, her condition, as Freud reported to Fliess, worsened: "...persistent swelling, going up and down 'like an avalanche'; pain, so that morphine cannot be dispensed with; bad nights ... [T]he day before yesterday (Saturday) she had a massive hemorrhage, probably as a result of expelling a bone chip the size of a heller [a coin]; there were two bowls full of pus."[81, p. 21]

A few days later, Freud wrote to Fliess that Emma had another nasal hemorrhage, which prompted Freud to take her to Ignaz Rosanes, a Viennese doctor, who:

> ...cleaned the area surrounding the opening, removed some sticky blood clots, and suddenly pulled at something like a thread, kept on pulling. Before either of us had time to think, at least half a meter of gauze had been removed from the cavity. The next moment came a flood of blood ... At the moment the foreign body came out and everything became clear to me—and I immediately afterward was confronted by the sight of the patient—I felt sick ... I do not believe it was the blood that overwhelmed me—at that moment strong emotions were welling up in me. So we had done her an injustice ... That this mishap should have happened to you ... [82, p. 22]

That Freud remarked to Fliess, "[W]e had done her an injustice" is to his credit. But that he shows more concern about Fliess's feelings—"That this mishap should have happened to you"—rather than about Emma is disappointing. Yet, commentators have remarked on how Freud and Fliess were becoming intoxicated with their psychological theories and, indeed, with one another. Mary Jane Lupton surmises that their meetings and correspondences "…showed strong signs of repressed homosexual desire,"[83, p. 18] so that Emma at best represents a vehicle by which the two physicians' relationship deepened. Fliess's failure to remove the gauze, however, and the fetid, putrid, foreign object it came to represent, had shaken Freud, who would have to resolve this medical error and the rupture that it threatened to his relationship with Fliess.

This Freud did by blaming Emma. In a letter to Fliess about a year after the incident, Freud made Emma out to be the guilty one, the one who desired to bleed: "Her hemorrhages were hysterical, brought on by longing, probably at the 'sexual period,'"[84, p. 23] that is, her menstrual period. In another letter to Fliess about a month later, Freud convinced himself that it did not matter whether Emma bled through her nose or through her vagina:

> I know only that she bled out of longing. She has always been a bleeder, when cutting herself and in similar circumstances; as a child she suffered from severe nosebleeds; during the years when she was not yet menstruating, she had headaches which were interpreted to her as malingering and which in truth had been generated by suggestion; for this reason she joyously welcomed her severe menstrual bleeding as proof that her illness was genuine.[85, p. 24]

And so the father of psychoanalysis, intent on preserving a warm professional relationship with a professional colleague, heady (and haughty?) with his germinating ideas on the sexual basis of the neuroses—*The Interpretation of Dreams* would appear in only four years—and pained, no doubt, by the wrong done his patient but about whose welfare, it appears, he never seemed entirely committed, solved his anxieties by making her take the blame for the affair. Emma's reaction to it all, incidentally, bears reporting: When the putrid gauze was removed and Freud appeared shaken, Emma—who remained conscious throughout the entire, ghastly procedure—is supposed to have looked at him and said sarcastically, "So this is the strong sex."[86, p. 23]

While I am unaware as to whether Emma realized Fliess's error, I can observe that the HIRP's (or FOT's) projection of superiority and authority may very well feel dismissive or distancing to many patients. As such, the HIRP is precisely the kind of health professional for whom error concealment tokens an immense liability risk. A harm-causing error that is concealed by the HIRP but then discovered by the harmed party is likely to trigger the latter's rage toward this aloof and arrogant individual. Just as the HIRP might prefer contractual relationships with patients and express profound displeasure if the patient fails to live up to his share of the terms, so that attitude will encourage the patient to feel similarly toward the HIRP. Should the HIRP default on his contractual obligation of rendering care according to the professional standard, the patient might indict the HIRP a fraud. Should the HIRP then proceed to explain the error deceptively, the patient might perceive the HIRP as evil.

Compulsiveness

Gabbard claimed that, "[T]here is no doubt that compulsiveness is the hallmark of the physician's personality" and that, "compulsive traits are present in the majority of those individuals who seek out medicine as a profession."[87, p. 2926] But if compulsiveness means paying keen and thoughtful attention to a patient's clinical situation, it clearly seems a desirable and especially an adaptive trait. Compulsiveness becomes pathological when it is driven by inordinately masochistic "super-ego" demands that are impossible to fulfill and that compromise important relationships with others.[88]

While compulsive people (COMPs) are often enormously successful at what they do and might even desire to establish caring relationships, their ideological rigidity, exacting standards, tendency to catastrophize, and lingering doubt that they have not covered every possible contingency tend to compromise their interpersonal relationships. The COMP's unhealthy narcissism exists in his or her immense fear of failure—a fear that is utterly unbearable because, like most narcissists, the idea of his or her being mediocre or average is intolerable.[89]

If health professionals are already inclined toward compulsiveness, a healthy sense of self-esteem becomes crucial in keeping their compulsiveness from compromising their interpersonal relationships. The emotionally unhealthy COMP exemplifies the overachieving, rather than high-achieving, narcissist and will probably have immense difficulties setting reasonable limits on his projects, aspirations, and expectations of others.[90] These more psychologically fragile individuals are acutely sensitive to feelings of guilt and doubt so they work immensely hard to keep the possibility of failure at bay, to appease their anxieties over unfinished business, and to accommodate their distorted self-understanding as indispensable. This kind of medical narcissist is nicely captured in one of Gabbard's vignettes:

> Dr. B was getting ready to leave his office at 6 PM to rush home and have supper before attending his son's final high school basketball game. The hospital called to inform him that one of his patients had arrived in labor and delivery and was currently showing 5 cm of cervical dilatation. He knew that one of his partners was covering that night but he felt compelled to run by the hospital to check her before going home. After checking her, he decided to stay through the delivery, necessitating his missing his son's last game.
>
> Afterwards, the physician wept. He could not understand why he had not simply handed the case over to his partner. He stated later that he was not even emotionally attached to this particular patient. His narcissism had gotten the best of him. He felt that he and he alone had to be the one to deliver the baby, as though his partner could not have performed exactly the same function.[91, p. 2928]

In this case, the physician's deep need to be at the center of what is happening, his discomfort over the thought of losing "his" patient to a colleague, and perhaps his need to be respected overwhelmed his feelings for his own family. Oddly, the physician did not personally care about this patient, yet he refused to leave the hospital and enjoy his son's final basketball game. What this physician attached a fundamental importance to was his own attentional needs, his anxiety that something might go wrong and that only he could correct the problem, his need to be in the spotlight and share the moment with his patient, and his need for the patient's gratitude. How could he possibly give all that up for a back seat in the bleachers with the spotlight turned on his son?

With their superiors, COMPs are often excessively polite, obedient, and deferential—possibly because such behaviors calm their anxieties about being entirely to blame if things go wrong. With their subordinates, COMPs with poor self-esteem are often obnoxiously demanding, uncompromising, and merciless in meting out reprimands and condemnations.[92]

A physician offered the following story of her bizarre encounter with such a person when she was in medical school. As a third-year medical student, she found herself on an elevator with a senior resident and with one of the attending physicians on the floor. The resident, who had missed morning rounds, asked the medical student a few questions about one of his patients, about whom the student knew next to nothing because the patient was not hers. After telling the resident she was not able to answer his questions, she went on:

> At that moment the attending stepped directly in front of my face and said "If you came from my medical school I would knock you to the floor and you'd be bleeding—and I would be a hero for that."[93, p. 136]

This extreme, and doubtlessly very rare, reaction shows the COMP at his (and in this case, because the attending physician was female, her) sadistic worst. As far as the attending was concerned, the student should have known everything about every patient in the unit, regardless of whether the patient was assigned to the student or not. The student's confession of ignorance provoked such anxiety that it triggered the attending's sadistic rage. As far as the attending was concerned, omniscience is a perfectly reasonable pedagogical expectation so that the student who fell short of it deserved to be bloodied.

The Compulsive's Reaction to Medical Error

The highly compulsive professional's perception of a serious medical error is probably marked by immense shock. If compulsiveness is indeed at the heart of the health professional's personality, the reports we saw in the previous chapter of health professionals' descriptions of their psychosomatic reactions to errors may well be representative. COMPs are very unlikely to casually dismiss a serious or, indeed, any kind of error. Psychologically fragile COMPs will either direct inordinate, and sometimes suicidal, hostility at themselves or vent their spleen at others. The undeniable medical error that the COMP commits is extremely painful evidence of what he has feared all of his life: worthlessness.[94]

Of the various kinds of narcissistic types discussed in this section, the COMP is least likely to dismiss error. Bertrand Russell is supposed to have said, "One of the symptoms of an approaching nervous breakdown is the belief that one's work is terribly important."[95, p. 528] The compulsive narcissist lives on that edge because he or she combines an exaggerated sense of responsibility with an exaggerated fear of failure with an exaggerated belief about his or her importance.[96] This results in the COMP having a hard time determining salience or priorities because every task becomes an extension of the COMP's exaggerated (i.e., narcissistic) self-formation. Indeed, stories are commonly told about physicians who, when they suspect another health professional, who is often a nurse, has committed an error, go immediately and directly to the patient and disclose it, rather than first going to hospital risk management to have the error investigated. Later on, it might be discovered that an error did not really occur, but by then any representation to the patient that tries to reinterpret the error into a non-error will be unconvincing.

If any of the various narcissistic types described in this chapter feel conflicted over disclosing an error to a harmed patient, however, it would be the COMP—not because he resonates with patient-centered rights, but because he feels unbearably guilty. Furthermore, it is unlikely that the COMP would disclose for the sake of receiving forgiveness, but rather because it would somehow feel right to suffer through a public statement of his or her wretchedness. *It ought not surprise us, then, that this "mea culpa" reaction of the COMP has been keenly recognized over the last century and been intercepted not by error disclosure to the harmed party but by that venerable institution, the morbidity and mortality conference.* Here, and behind closed doors, physicians confess certain of their errors to one another, receive professional rebuke, and perhaps absolution. As Charles Bosk pointed out in his famous book *Forgive and Remember,* the morbidity and mortality conference serves as a "hair-shirt" ritual, whereby error perpetrators confess their sins, humble themselves before their peers, and hope that they receive forgiveness and be reabsorbed back into the fold.[97] Yet, the fact that this ritual occurs not in front of the patients they have harmed but rather in front of their peers tends to reinforce the narcissistic insularity of physicians and encourages their belief that errors can be managed internally and need not be comprehensively disclosed.

Although they can drive everybody crazy and cause an unprecedented degree of burnout, psychologically fragile COMPS are pitiful. Not only does their narcissism incline them to think that their agenda and convictions are supremely important (and so they exploit people in completing that agenda), but COMPs also find themselves in the midst of an ever-expanding, self-generated swamp of details, processes, and informational glut that they nevertheless believe requires exhaustive attention to avert catastrophe. But the number of variables that can compromise success is immense and no human being can adequately manage them all. COMPs implicitly know this, which is why their affect—rather unlike other narcissistic types—is typically one of edginess, depression, or frustration.[98] When it comes to medical errors, the COMP may well be a loose cannon who identifies errors where there are none, holds himself and everyone else to an impossible level of accountability, impulsively rather than thoughtfully responds to error accusations, and generally misconstrues the meaning of error—such as in his or her meting out inordinate blame rather than examining the error's systemic causes and working on his or her empathic skills. Given these inclinations, the COMP's response to error is unlikely to foster healthy relationships or advance patient safety, while it would not be unusual for serious harm to result from the COMP's own psychological unraveling.

Conclusion

Given the emotional tsunami that health professionals routinely experience in their training, one can only marvel at how so many of them—indeed, probably the majority—come through relatively psychologically intact. Consider how students and freshly minted professionals must withstand a daily frontal attack on their self-esteem and psychological equilibrium that is punctuated by their obvious clinical ignorance as beginners; their powerlessness in being lowest on the hierarchical totem pole; their almost hourly confrontation with performance anxiety that is further aggravated by their need to get a good grade or evaluation; their intense desire to be a part of a team whose rules of inclusiveness they do not yet understand; and an ongoing exposure to the occasionally immense pain and misery of other human beings to whom they are professionally obligated. Stereotypically, as students they are profoundly caring and compassionate, but they inevitably observe certain of their teachers engaging in morally problematic patient interactions. Furthermore, all of this occurs against a backdrop of an immensely complex operational environment that usually runs at a less than optimal mode and in which mistakes, confusion, ambiguous communications, technological breakdowns, and unclear lines of authority abound.

Regardless of whether one is a flamboyant, exhibitionistic narcissist, or quietly harbors fantasies of grandeur that he or she takes pains to conceal, or is constantly fighting off feelings of inadequacy and worthlessness that have been part of his or her psychological formation since childhood, narcissistic behaviors ultimately offer a refuge from anxiety over one's respectability and self-esteem. The extreme narcissist goes through life with a psychological armor that nothing can penetrate. These persons will never achieve self-understanding because their psychological formation prevents them from differentiating their image in Narcissus's pool from their real self. Intoxicated by their narcissism—indeed, these people literally get "drunk" rhapsodizing about themselves—their self-understanding stops with their image in the pool. They *are* that image. Other, and indeed most, unhealthy narcissists are not nearly so absolute in their sense of self. Their narcissism exists side by side with painful feelings of insecurity and self-doubt that trigger their narcissistic behaviors.

While the healthy narcissist might be crestfallen by the occasional failure, he or she will retain a sensitivity toward others; a reasonable degree of objectivity about his or her accomplishments and those of others; a feeling of self-confidence while nevertheless being cognizant of his or her flaws and imperfections; and an authentic sense of humility in the face of life's challenges, miseries, and tragedies. Thus, the "healthy" medical narcissist will engage the patient in comprehensive informed consent discussions. He or she will take pains to ensure that the patient understands this information, and supportively corrects any misunderstandings or unrealistic fantasies the patient might harbor. Most important, if the risks or burdens disclosed in the consent process materialize, this health professional will not argue with or dismiss the patient's feelings, but will assist the patient to find the support he or she needs to manage a clinical disappointment. The unhealthy medical narcissist, however, will find these kinds of patient interactions very difficult going, indeed.

Because unhealthy narcissism often attempts to deny or repress all that healthy narcissism admits, Howard Spiro's comment that "physicians are trained in narcissism" gives pause as to how narcissism develops not only in individual personalities but in healthcare cultures. We have seen how narcissism can ameliorate feelings of inadequacy, and few experiences in healthcare conjure up such feelings as those connected with a serious harm-causing error. The next chapter offers a case study that illustrates how these self-protective narcissistic proclivities especially result in avoidance reactions to the discomfort of error disclosure.

References

1. Berger, Thomas. *Vital Parts*. Quoted in *The 2,548 Best Things Anybody Ever Said*, ed. Robert Byrne, New York: Simon & Schuster, 2003.

2. Spiro, Howard M. "What is empathy and can it be taught?" In *Empathy and the Practice of Medicine*, eds. Howard M. Spiro, Mary G. McRea Curnen, Enid Peschel, and Deborah St. James. New Haven: Yale University Press, 1993, pp. 7–14.

3. Gabbard, Glen O., and Menninger, Roy W. "The psychology of the physician." In *Medical Marriages*, eds. Glen O. Gabbard and Roy W. Menninger. Washington, DC: American Psychiatric Press, 1988, pp. 23–38.

4. Cloninger, C. Robert, and Svrakic, Dragan M. "Personality disorders." In *Kaplan & Sadock's Comprehensive Textbook of Psychiatry, Volume II, Seventh Edition*, eds. Benjamin J. Sadock and Virginia Sadock. Philadelphia: Lippincott Williams & Wilkins, 2000, pp. 1723–1764 (see especially 1745–1746); also see Gorton, Gregg E. "Personality disorders." In *Clinical Psychiatry for Medical Students*, 3rd Edition, ed. Alan Stoudemire, Philadelphia: Lippincott-Raven, 1998, pp. 186–241; and Allnutt, S., and Links, P. S. "Diagnosing specific personality disorders and the optimal criteria." In *Clinical Assessment and Management of Severe Personality Disorders*, ed. P. S. Links. Washington, DC: American Psychiatric Press, 1996, pp. 21–47, at 36.

5. Masterson, James F. *The Search for the Real Self*. New York: The Free Press, 1988.

6. Watson, Paul J.; Hickman, Susan E.; Morris, Ronald J.; Milliron, J. Trevor; and Whiting, Linda. "Narcissism, self-esteem, and parental nurturance." *The Journal of Psychology*. 129(1):61–73, 1995. For a list of publications, see the references at the end of this paper.

7. Watson et al., 1995.

8. Masterson, 1988.

9. Stone, Michael. "Etiology of borderline personality disorder: Psychobiological factors contributing to an underlying irritability." Quoted in Millon, Theodore. *Disorder of Personality: DSM-IV and Beyond*. New York: John Wiley & Sons, Inc., 1996.

10. Winnicott, Donald W. *The Maturational Processes and the Facilitating Environment*. New York: International Universities Press, 1965.

11. Kernberg, Otto. "An ego psychology object relations theory of the structure and treatment of pathologic narcissism: An overview." In Kernberg, 1989. Kohut, Heinz. *Restoration of the Self*. New York: International Universities Press, 1977. For a more readable account of Kohut, see Goldberg, Arnold. "Self-psychology and the narcissistic personality disorders." In Kernberg, 1989, pp. 731–739.

12. Kernberg, 1989.

13. Masterson, 1988.

14. Akhtar, Salman. "Narcissistic personality disorder: Descriptive features and differential diagnosis." In *Narcissistic Personality Disorder. Psychiatric Clinics of North America*, ed. Otto Kernberg, 12(3):505–529, 1989.

15. Masterson, 1988.

16. Miller, Alice. *The Drama of the Gifted Child*. New York: Basic Books, 1997.

17. Miller, 1997.

18. Masterson, 1988.

19. Masterson, 1988.

20. Kernberg, 1989.

21. In a telephone conversation, Dr. Hedberg related to this author that he believes he got the "12 Step Program" from the Internet, but that he has been unable to locate it again. Further attempts to locate its origins have proved unsuccessful.

22. Epstein, Mark. *Thoughts without a Thinker*. New York: Basic Books, 1995.

23. Gabbard and Menninger, 1988.

24. Gabbard and Menninger, 1988.

25. Epstein, 1995.

26. Gabbard and Menninger, 1988.

27. Vaillant, George E.; Sobowale, Nancy Corbin; and McArthur, Charles. "Some psychologic vulnerabilities of physicians." *New England Journal of Medicine.* 287(8):372–375, 1972.

28. Misch, Donald A. "Evaluating physicians' professionalism and humanism: The case for humanism 'connoisseurs.'" *Academic Medicine.* 77(6):489–495, 2002.

29. Misch, 2002.

30. Gabbard, Glen O. "The role of compulsiveness in the normal physician." *JAMA.* 254(20):2926–2929, 1985.

31. Robins, Lynne S.; Braddock, Clarence H. III; and Fryer-Edwards, Kelly A. "Using the American Board of Internal Medicine's 'Elements of Professionalism'" for undergraduate ethics education." *Academic Medicine.* 77(6):523–531, 2002.

32. Watson, Paul J.; Hickman, Susan E.; and Morris, Ronald J. "Self-reported narcissism and shame: Testing the defensive self-esteem and continuum hypotheses." *Personality and Individual Differences.* 21(2):253–259, 1996; Watson, Paul J.; Morris, Ronald J.; and Miller, Liv. "Narcissism and the self as continuum: Correlations with assertiveness and hypercompetitiveness." *Imagination, Cognition and Personality.* 17(3):249–259, 1997–98; Watson, Paul J.; Varnell, Sherri P.; and Morris, Ronald J. "Self-reported narcissism and perfectionism: An ego-psychological perspective and the continuum hypothesis. "*Imagination, Cognition and Personality.* 19(1):59–69, 2000.

33. Maxmin, J. S. "Do we hear our patients? And would a patient's page help?" *BMJ.* 324(16 March):684, 2002.

34. Branch, William; Pels, Richard J.; Lawrence, Robert S.; and Arky, Ronald. "Becoming a doctor: Critical-incident reports from third year medical students." *New England Journal of Medicine.* 329(15):1130–1132, 1993.

35. This author bases these estimates on interviews with Emory medical students and medical school admissions staff.

36. Leichtman, Martin. "The occupational hazards of having a physician father." In *Medical Marriages,* eds. Glen O. Gabbard and Roy Menninger, 1988, pp. 103–119.

37. Leichtman, 1988.

38. Leichtman, 1988.

39. Leichtman, 1988.

40. Leichtman, 1988.

41. Leichtman, 1988.

42. Duncan, David Ewing. *Residents: The Perils and Promise of Educating Young Doctors.* New York: Scribner, 1996.

43. Benner, Patricia; Tanner, Christine; and Chesla, Catherine. *Expertise in Nursing Practice: Caring, Clinical Judgment, and Ethics.* New York: Springer, 1996.

44. Benner, Tanner, and Chesla, 1996.

45. Benner, Tanner, and Chesla, 1996.

46. Feudtner, Chris, and Christakis, Dimitri A. "Making the rounds: The ethical development of medical students in the context of clinical rotations." *Hastings Center Report.* 24(1):6–12, 1994.

47. Feudtner, Chris; Christakis, Dimitri A.; and Christakis, Nicholas A. "Do clinical clerks suffer ethical erosion? Students' perceptions of their ethical environment and personal development." *Academic Medicine.* 68(8):670–679, 1994; Daugherty, Steven R.; Baldwin, DeWitt C. Jr.; and Rowley, Beverley D. "Learning, satisfaction, and mistreatment during medical internship: A national survey of working conditions." *JAMA.* 279(15):1194–1199, 1998. Baldwin, DeWitt C. Jr.; Daugherty, Steven R.; and Rowley, Beverley D. "Unethical and unprofessional conduct observed by residents during their first year of training." *Academic Medicine.* 73(11):1195–1200, 1998; Sheehan, K. Harnett; Sheehan, David V.; White, Kim; Leibowitz, Alan; and Baldwin, DeWitt C. "A pilot study of medical student 'abuse': Student perceptions of mistreatment and misconduct in medical school." *JAMA.* 263(4):533–537, 1990.

48. Spiro, 1993.

49. Duncan, 1996.

50. McCall, Timothy. "The impact of long working hours on resident physicians." *New England Journal of Medicine.* 318(12):775–778, 1988.

51. Duncan, 1996.

52. Duncan, 1996.

53. Duncan, 1996.

54. Gabbard and Menninger, 1988.

55. Duncan, 1996.

56. Marcus, Eric. "Empathy, humanism, and the professionalization process of medical education." *Academic Medicine.* 74(11):1211–1215, 1999.

57. Duncan, 1996.

58. Papers from which I learned much about projection are: Gunther, Meyer. "Catastrophic illness and the caregivers: Real burdens and solutions with respect to the role of the behavioral sciences." In *Rehabilitation Psychology Desk Reference*, ed. Bruce Caplan, Rockville, MD: Aspen, 1987, pp. 219–243; Gans, Jerome. "Facilitating staff/patient interaction in rehabilitation." In Caplan, 1987, pp. 185–218. The best collection of papers on projection (which is a type of transference) that this author has come across is in Robert Lang's anthology, *Classics in Psychoanalytic Technique.* Northvale, NJ: Aronson, 1990. The most gripping account of projection I have ever read is Maltsburger, J.T., and Buie, D.H. "Countertransference hate in the treatment of suicidal patients." *Archives of General Psychiatry.* 30(5):625–633, 1974.

59. *Between a Rock and Hard Place: Values, Ethics, and the Physician-In-Training: Salvage Chemotherapy.* A videotape created by the American Medical Student

Association Standing Committee on Bioethics. Grant support provided by E. R. Squibb and Sons, Inc., Henry J. Kaiser Family Foundation, and the Department of Internal Medicine, Stanford University School of Medicine.

60. Berger, Allan. "Arrogance among physicians." *Academic Medicine.* 77(2): 145–147, 2002.

61. Osler, William. *The Collected Essays of Sir William Osler, Vol 1. The Philosophical Essays.* Edited and with an introduction by John P. McGovern and Charles Roland. Birmingham, AL: The Classics Modern Library, 1985.

62. Osler, 1985.

63. Halpern, Jodi. *From Detached Concern to Empathy: Humanizing Medical Practice.* Oxford, UK: Oxford University Press, 2001.

64. Halpern, 2001.

65. Katz, Pearl. *The Scalpel's Edge: The Culture of Surgeons.* Boston, MA: Allyn and Bacon, 1999.

66. Mahler-Werfels, Alma. *And the Bridge Is Love.* New York: Harcourt, Brace and Company, 1958.

67. Levinson, Wendy, and Chaumeton, Nigel. "Communication between surgeons and patients in routine office visits." *Surgery.* 125(2):127–134, 1999.

68. Macciocchi, Stephen N., and Eaton, Bradford. "Decision and attribution bias in neurorehabilitation." *Archives of Physical Medicine and Rehabilitation.* 76(6):521–524, 1995.

69. Macciocchi and Eaton, 1995.

70. Gunther, 1987.

71. Christensen, John F.; Levinson, Wendy; and Dunn, Patrick M. "The heart of darkness: The impact of perceived mistakes on physicians," *Journal of General Internal Medicine* 7 (July/August): 424–431, 1992; Hickson, Gerald B.; Clayton, Ellen Wright; Githens, Penny B.; and Sloan, Frank A. "Factors that prompted families to file medical malpractice claims following perinatal injuries." *JAMA.* 267(10):1359–1363, 1992; Finkelstein, Daniel; Wu, Albert W.; Holtzman, Neil A.; and Smith, Melanie K. "When a physician harms a patient by a medical error: Ethical, legal and risk-management considerations," *The Journal of Clinical Ethics* 8(4): 330–335, 1997.

72. Gallagher, Thomas H.; Waterman, Amy D.; Ebers, Alison G.; Fraser, Victoria J.; and Levinson, Wendy. "Patients' and physicians attitudes regarding the disclosure of medical errors." *JAMA.* 289(8):1001–1007, 2003.

73. Gunther, 1987.

74. Masterson, 1988.

75. A wonderful example of this is Anne Fadiman's *The Spirit Catches You and You Fall Down.* New York: Farrar, Straus and Giroux, 1997.

76. Halpern, 2001.

77. Rubin, Jane. "Impediments to the development of clinical knowledge and ethical judgment in critical care nursing." In Benner, Tanner, and Chesla, 1996, pp. 170–192.

78. Childress, James. *Practical Reasoning in Bioethics*. Bloomington, IN: Indiana University Press, 1997.

79. Lupton, Mary Jane. *Menstruation and Psychoanalysis*. Urbana, IL: University of Illinois Press, 1993.

80. Lupton, 1993.

81. Lupton, 1993.

82. Lupton, 1993.

83. Lupton, 1993.

84. Lupton, 1993.

85. Lupton, 1993.

86. Lupton, 1993.

87. Gabbard, 1985.

88. Gabbard, 1985.

89. Readers wishing a technically elaborate account of pathologic compulsiveness can consult Theodore Millon's *Disorders of Personality*, 1996, pp. 505–539. A highly readable and entertaining account of both the narcissist and compulsive personalities can be found in Albert J. Bernstein. *Emotional Vampires: Dealing with People Who Drain You Dry*. New York: McGraw Hill, 2001.

90. Millon, 1996; Bernstein, 2001.

91. Gabbard, 1985.

92. Millon, 1996; Bernstein, 2001.

93. Kushner, Thomasine K., and Thomasma, David C. (eds). *Ward Ethics: Dilemmas for Medical Students and Doctors in Training*. Cambridge, UK: Cambridge University Press, 2001.

94. Millon, 1996; Bernstein, 2001.

95. Rosten, Leo (ed.). *Carnival of Wit*. New York: Penguin Books, 1996.

96. Gabbard, 1985.

97. Bosk, Charles. *Forgive and Remember*. Chicago, IL: The University of Chicago Press, 1979.

98. Millon, 1996; Bernstein, 2001.

Chapter 4

SCRAM:
A Case Study

"[W]e were beginning to really be suspect, when—when people treat you like you're radio-active material ... We need to know what the heck's going on here, and it—it's like it was falling on deaf ears."
Family member whose mother experienced medical error commenting on lack of communication

Introduction

T he preceding chapters suggest that the occurrence of a serious, harm-causing medical error frequently triggers various psychological reactions among the involved health professionals, which can then encourage the withholding of information about the error from the harmed parties. In some instances, that information might be utterly concealed, while in others, and probably most, the information might be disclosed in a way that does not call attention to or admit the error, or that does not incriminate the professionals involved in the error's commission.

The argument of this book is that a primary source of these avoidance reactions to error and its disclosure is a mix of very unpleasant psychological reactions compounded by a kind of medical "narcissism." An advanced narcissism might cause certain health professionals to deny, dismiss, or ignore the error completely, as their self-comprehension as perfect or never-erring precludes them from admitting responsibility for the error or its harm. A more common narcissistically based reaction to error, and one that we will see in the case study below, is one that looks to avoidance and denial strategies to protect the health professional from the anxiety associated with disclosing the error. In these instances, an error might indeed be admitted by and among the treating professionals along with the possibility that it caused harm. Yet, because medical errors occur in the midst of environments that are technologically and psychosocially complex, different persons might interpret or explain what happened, why it happened, and what it ultimately means in immensely different ways, largely depending on how their own self-interests will fare per the information disclosed. The point of this chapter, and indeed of this book, is to explore how those self-interests can compromise the health professionals' moral obligation of disclosure when a serious harm-causing error occurred.

The preceding chapters show that the occurrence of a serious, harm-causing medical error often triggers an intense feeling of shock combined immediately with anxious feelings of concern. The first object of concern is usually for the welfare of the harmed party, while the second is for the welfare of the erring professional. As these concerns and their accompanying anxieties are played out, many health professionals will naturally seek tension-relieving strategies. The objective of these strategies will be to avoid precisely what moral reflection and action require, namely, confronting the reality of the error and its consequences in a patient-centered way. As we saw in the second chapter, avoidance can be effected by a host of rationalizations that reinterpret the scenario as non-errant or harmless, or that deflect responsibility away from the error operators. If these rationalizing strategies are successful, they will result in the health professional's having minimized the error, its harm, or his or her responsibility for it. But, if the health professional attempts to offer his or her rationalized version of what occurred to the harmed party, that communication might well strike the listener as dismissive and even deceptive, because the listener will want truthful information delivered in a way that acknowledges his or her own pain and sense of outrage. A professional's rationalizing or minimizing response will accomplish just the opposite.

Shock, concern, rationalization, avoidance, and minimization offer the acronym SCRAM. We will now turn to an actual case study that illustrates the elements of this acronym and what might be learned from them. The material that is presented below is taken entirely from a malpractice action with which I have been professionally involved. To protect the privacy of everyone concerned, I will simply refer to the physicians who played roles in this case as Dr. Anesthesiologist, Dr. Surgeon, et cetera. I will call the patient who was harmed Mrs. Betty Smith, her adult daughter Patty Smith, and her adult son, Michael Smith. All of the material that is presented as quotations is taken virtually verbatim from the individuals' sworn depositions.

The Case

Beginning approximately at 10:45 AM on a Monday, Betty Smith, an otherwise healthy and vigorous 62-year-old woman, underwent elective, upper abdominal surgery. About an hour into the procedure, the surgeon requested that the anesthesiologist turn off the ventilator for a few seconds so that an X-ray of Mrs. Smith's abdomen could be taken without movement artifact (which is a common request). The anesthesiologist, who had been administering oxygen at a concentration of 50 percent, turned the toggle switch of the ventilator to the "off" position and then, after a few seconds, thought that he flipped the switch back to "on." Because the X-ray cassette for the picture had apparently gotten stuck in its slot and because the surgical table had been raised for the imaging procedure but was now resisting being lowered because of a stuck gear, the anesthesiologist got up from his station to assist. He then returned to his work station whereupon, after an unspecified period of time that could have been anywhere from a few to as many as 30 minutes, he noticed that the ventilator was in the "off" position. As was later revealed in various depositions, all the anesthesia monitoring alarms had apparently been programmed to a "suspend indefinite" mode or were turned off. Once aware that the ventilator was off, Dr. Anesthesiologist immediately switched it to "on" and increased the oxygen concentration to 100 percent but did not tell the surgeon. The operation concluded around 12:45 PM. When Mrs. Smith failed to awaken from surgery and was unable to be extubated and breathe without ventilatory support, the surgeon was called and had a brief discussion with the anesthesiologist in the post-operative recovery room. It was at that time, about 90 minutes after the surgery was completed, that the anesthesiologist told the surgeon about the ventilator being off for an unspecified period. At her deposition, the surgeon testified that she informed Mrs. Smith's neurologist and pulmonologist of the error that very afternoon, since they would be caring for her in the intensive care unit to which she was transferred.

At their depositions, both the neurologist and pulmonologist testified that they informed the hospital's administration of the error by the following morning.

Mrs. Smith never awoke from surgery and remained on a ventilator. Within a few days following surgery, she was diagnosed as being in a persistent vegetative state with globally anoxic brain damage. On Tuesday of the following week, Mrs. Smith's family consented to her being disconnected from the ventilator, and she died approximately 48 hours later. During Mrs. Smith's hospitalization, her family was never informed of the ventilator accident that was, in all likelihood, the cause of her catastrophic neurological injury. The Smith family learned about the error after they secured legal assistance and an investigation uncovered the error.

Shock and Concern

For the patient. Michael Smith met Dr. Anesthesiologist within an hour after his mother's operation. At that time, Michael had no idea there was a problem with his mother's surgery until Dr. Anesthesiologist told him that his mother was "not coming out of the anesthesia as quickly as we would like her to." Michael went on to say that:

> It struck me that he was extremely nervous … He was red in the face. He was sweating, having a hard time making eye contact. Of course, I didn't know if maybe he'd just got out of surgery and was hot from the operating room. But it struck me that he was very nervous, and he immediately started apologizing. He said I'm sorry.

Although Dr. Anesthesiologist admitted at his deposition that at some point around 11:45 AM the ventilator was off for an indeterminate period, he never charted the absence of ventilation for Mrs. Smith in his anesthesia record. When he discovered that the ventilator was off, Dr. Anesthesiologist claimed that he switched from giving Mrs. Smith 50 percent oxygen, which he had been doing from the beginning of the operation, to 100 percent oxygen. Still, he failed to chart the higher oxygen concentration as well and completed his entries only after the operation concluded. Although his failure to chart certain of these events might be explained as Dr. Anesthesiologist's not wanting to incriminate himself or admit liability in the medical record, Dr. Anesthesiologist's own explanation at deposition was that:

> [O]nce I discovered that Mrs. Smith's ventilator was off, I don't really remember—I don't know when I charted the rest of that. I mean, I was not—charting wasn't anything I was concerned with ... I was paying attention to Mrs. Smith and really not paying attention to the record.

In explaining why he waited 90 minutes after the operation to inform Dr. Surgeon of the ventilator problem, Dr. Anesthesiologist said: "My primary concern, at that particular time, was with Mrs. Smith and watching her respirations, monitoring her every second. And that was what I was concerned with."

Although Dr. Surgeon informed both the neurologist and pulmonologist who took over Mrs. Smith's care later that day of the ventilator error, Dr. Surgeon did not report Dr. Anesthesiologist to hospital administration for leaving the ventilator off until some weeks after Mrs. Smith's death. When asked why she waited so long, Dr. Surgeon replied:

> Because at that point [i.e., while Mrs. Smith was still alive] ... it was critical in this patient's management that the main thing that I was—I was concerned with and the main thing that I wanted was that this patient was taken care of in the most appropriate way, and the issues of filing a report and an incident report and dealing with administrative issues were not secondary but thirdly on my mind.

For oneself. While there is no doubt that Dr. Surgeon and Dr. Anesthesiologist were extremely upset over what happened, when Dr. Surgeon initially met with Patty Smith before the full extent of Mrs. Smith's injury became obvious, Patty remembers her saying:

> [Y]our mom's not waking up like—like—as expected. She said, "But first of all, you have to understand, I don't have any—I don't have any control of everything that goes on in surgery." She said, "That needs to be known right here." And, I mean, it just kind of hit us kind of odd.

A short time later, when Patty and Michael first visited their mother in the intensive care unit and were horrified to watch her thrashing and lunging about in bed and struggling with her endotracheal tube, Patty called Dr. Surgeon and asked if she had seen her mother. Patty remembered that, "She says 'Yes,' and then, she said to me, 'You are not going to pin this on me.'"

The first (and only) formal meeting that Dr. Anesthesiologist and Dr. Surgeon had with Michael and Patty Smith occurred on Wednesday night, over 50 hours after Mrs. Smith's surgery. In his deposition, Michael testified that, "Dr. Surgeon initiated the meeting by once again clarifying the point that she had no responsibility over the anesthesia administration nor [the] monitoring of it, and that struck me as pretty—pretty odd. Throw your own colleague under the bus here real fast like." And here is Patty Smith's description of Dr. Anesthesiologist at that meeting:

> Dr. Anesthesiologist actually said very little ... He was very nervous, very, very nervous ... He didn't look at us ... He was looking at the ground and shuffling his feet a lot, kind of rocking back and forth on his feet, moving his head back and forth, not looking at us.

In his deposition, Dr. Anesthesiologist did not express any moral appreciation for the Smith family's right to know what happened, either because he was mortified over the potential legal repercussions from such a revelation, or because he refused to believe, with any reasonable degree of certainty, that the ventilator error caused Mrs. Smith's brain insult. When he was asked at deposition, "Do you accept today that Mrs. Smith suffered global brain—a global brain injury as a result of oxygen deprivation during the surgical procedure?" Dr. Anesthesiologist responded, "I don't know the answer to that." When he was asked, "In your opinion, was it negligence for you to fail to turn the ventilator back on?" he said, "I'm not going to answer that question."

Although Michael and Patty Smith were never told of the error by any of the professionals treating their mother, we might note that when Dr. Pulmonologist and Dr. Neurologist were informed by Dr. Surgeon of the ventilator problem a few hours after Mrs. Smith's surgery, both of them reported the error to hospital administration in less than 24 hours.

Rationalization and Avoidance

During his deposition, Dr. Anesthesiologist seemed largely free of rationalizing over what happened. He even admitted at one point that the ventilator problem *could* have caused Mrs. Smith's anoxic injury, but he adamantly refused to say that it *did*. Perhaps Dr. Anesthesiologist convinced himself that the actual cause of Mrs. Smith's brain insult would never be known with absolute certainty—which, in itself, would be true—and that, therefore, his confessing ignorance as to its etiology was, in fact, truthful.

Nevertheless, Dr. Anesthesiologist seemed the arch avoider: He avoided charting that the ventilator was turned off; he avoided informing the surgeon until an hour and a half after the operation of the ventilator error; he avoided the attorney's question as to whether he should have noticed the ventilator was off or whether it was negligence to leave the ventilator off for however long it was off; and he not only avoided informing the Smiths of the error, but he submitted a bill for his services.

Dr. Surgeon offered an interesting description of Dr. Anesthesiologist's initial admission that there was a ventilator problem. When she was asked when was the first time that Dr. Anesthesiologist informed her that he had forgotten to turn the ventilator back on, Dr. Surgeon replied:

> You know, I'm not exactly sure, but his—his kind of thrust or his tone was of reassurance that he thinks that she's going to be okay ... [H]is kind of

comment wasn't that he had forgotten anything, but it was more like, you know, "The patient was off the vent for a while, but I think she's going to be okay." And I think that that's really the comment that was—most sticks in my mind.

One wonders what to make of this. Was Dr. Anesthesiologist in the throes of denial that anything harmful could befall Mrs. Smith? Was he fantasizing that, "he hadn't forgotten anything"? Was he unconsciously trying to shift blame to Mrs. Smith by saying, "the patient was off the vent for a while"—that she was somehow to blame for this?

Perhaps, though, Dr. Anesthesiologist and Dr. Surgeon rationalized their withholding information about the ventilator problem by way of a partial or half-truth admission, as described in a previous chapter. That is, during the Wednesday night conversation that Dr. Anesthesiologist and Dr. Surgeon conducted with the Smith family, Patty Smith distinctly recalled Dr. Surgeon saying, "her [mother's] brain was completely without oxygen. She said she was without oxygen." Nevertheless, according to Patty Smith's testimony, Dr. Surgeon and Dr. Anesthesiologist then followed that true statement with a lie. Patty recalled asking Dr. Surgeon and Dr. Anesthesiologist:

> "[D]o you have any idea when that was?" [i.e., her mother being without oxygen.] "No, I don't know." I said, "Well, could it possibly have been during surgery?" "I don't know." I said, "Well, could it have been during recovery?" "I just don't know."

In retrospect and assuming Patty Smith's recollection is accurate, pressuring Drs. Surgeon and Anesthesiologist at the Wednesday night meeting as to how her mother could have been without oxygen constituted the moment when Dr. Surgeon and Dr. Anesthesiologist could have taken the moral high ground. Had the physicians summoned the requisite courage and told the Smiths of the ventilator problem—or had they met the family again some days later when the ventilator problem by then seemed the only explanation for what happened to their mother and told them—it is extremely unlikely that this case would have taken the anguishing road it did. As it was, the Smiths remembered the physicians' confession of ignorance as to what caused their mother's brain damage as a lie. In a series of questions Patty was asked at her deposition, she said:

> *Patty:* I think his [i.e., the anesthesiologist's] license should go because he lied to me ...
>
> *Attorney:* Let me make certain that I understand. You are angry with Dr. Anesthesiologist because you believe he lied to you?
>
> *Patty:* Yes. Because I asked him point blank "When did it happen? Was she completely without air, or was she just laying there breathing or not breathing good enough for a long time?" "I don't know." That is a lie. And if you ask me, not telling somebody something is a lie.

What Dr. Anesthesiologist lacked in rationalizing capacity, however, was more than made up for by Dr. Surgeon. The fact that Mrs. Smith had apparently had a mini-stroke

10 years earlier, from which she completely recovered, nevertheless gave Dr. Surgeon considerable reason to believe, at least initially, that her brain injury was due to stroke. Indeed, Dr. Surgeon turned the word "stroke" into an etiological euphemism at the Wednesday night meeting. According to Patty Smith, Dr Surgeon said:

> [P]ossibly she's had another stroke. And I said … now generally when you have a stroke, I said, is it not generally just one side of your body or a portion or portions? And she said … "When I use the term 'stroke,' I—a drowning victim technically has had a stroke."

Michael Smith remembered something of the same: "We were going back and forth between a conversation about lack of oxygen and stroke, and then Dr. Surgeon explained that they were really one and the same."

At her deposition, Dr. Surgeon enumerated other differential diagnoses for Mrs. Smith including pulmonary edema, an air embolus, cardiac arrest, and the possibility of fatty tissue "storing" the anesthesia and slowing its release from Mrs. Smith's body. Dr. Surgeon also took solace in the fact that, "You don't know for sure in your own heart of hearts" as to what caused Mrs. Smith's brain damage, which seemed to relieve her from having to speculate about the possibility that the ventilator error was the proximate cause of Mrs. Smith's brain insult. Her rationalizations seemed to very much accommodate the observation made in Chapter 2 that rationalizations typify attempts to make weaker arguments or explanations triumph over stronger ones.

Yet, as the days following the surgery went by, Dr. Surgeon had to admit that these etiologic candidates she had been pinning her hopes on were less and less convincing. As Dr. Neurologist would later observe, the ventilator error "was the only story there was." And at her deposition Dr. Surgeon was asked:

> *Attorney:* And you came to understand that it was Dr. Anesthesiologist, through a lapse of attention to monitoring the patient and the state of her ventilation, that caused this tragedy; isn't that true?
>
> *Dr. Surgeon:* You know it—as the days went on, it seemed that that was the case.

When Dr. Surgeon was asked why, as the days following Mrs. Smith's surgery passed, she did not question Dr. Anesthesiologist more at length about what happened, she offered a reason that corroborated what was discussed earlier on the health professional's inclination to avoid anxiety-filled situations:

> You know, all I can tell you … is that I didn't, and I'm not sure why I didn't, and maybe one of the reasons why I didn't, if you want me to speculate, was that I was feeling so lousy about the whole thing and that I didn't want to bring it up … [W]hen something like this happens and you feel really terrible about it, you really don't like to talk about it … And I felt sick about this, and I really didn't want to talk about it.

Buttressing Dr. Surgeon's avoidance, however, was her continued ability to dismiss or deflect her moral responsibility to effect a disclosure of the error, such as in the following example where, in Golemanesque fashion, Dr. Surgeon fixed her attention on the clinical hopelessness of Betty Smith's condition and ignored whatever therapeutic value and moral respect error disclosure might have for Betty's family:

> [Y]ou're dealing with a situation that won't change the outcome of a very tragic event. There is nothing that we could have done to bring that lady's life back, and that's primarily the reason why I think this [i.e., disclosure] wasn't done.

Ultimately, Dr. Surgeon would plead that she did not disclose the ventilator problem and did not insist that Dr. Anesthesiologist do so because:

> I didn't want to go beyond what I knew for exact fact … in my own heart of hearts, I can't make someone tell something that he knows and that I'm just speculating about. Why as a man didn't he [i.e., Dr. Anesthesiologist] step up to the plate? How can I make him say something that I don't know for sure?

Interestingly, Dr. Neurologist and Dr. Pulmonologist used exactly this "distancing" or "degree of separation" excuse to explain why they did not effect a truthful disclosure of the ventilator problem to the Smith family. Both pleaded the unreliability of their "hearsay" knowledge of the error as it was relayed to them by Dr. Surgeon, and both believed that they dispatched whatever moral obligation they had to the Smith family by disclosing to hospital administration what Dr. Surgeon told them about the ventilator problem. Indeed, Dr. Neurologist admitted at his deposition that his office received a phone call from Dr. Anesthesiologist some days after the surgery, which he refused to return. When asked why, Dr. Neurologist responded:

> I don't know Dr. Anesthesiologist. I felt that it was not going to alter what I was going to do. I felt it may just confuse the issue for me as the neurologist who was taking care of the patient.

When he was explicitly asked if the real reason he did not return the call was because he thought Mrs. Smith's brain injury resulted from the ventilator problem, Dr. Neurologist answered, "No."

Taking Pause

Allow me to pause here for a moment and point out that all of the above was gleaned from the principals' depositions and therefore constitutes a recollected reconstruction of what the first few days were like for them following Mrs. Smith's surgery. In defense of Drs. Surgeon, Anesthesiologist, Neurologist, and Pulmonologist, we might remark that in the first few days following Mrs. Smith's surgery, it was probably entirely appropriate for them to proceed to hospital administration and rely on the organization's management of the error. Drs. Neurologist and Pulmonologist's going directly to administration and revealing what they knew about the error is sound operational and moral policy since one can truthfully say that in the first 48 or so hours following Mrs. Smith's surgery, there was *no reasonable degree of certainty* that the ventilator error was responsible or would be responsible for her brain insult. The extent of Mrs. Smith's injury was unknown at that time while Drs. Pulmonologist and Neurologist did not have access to any documentation about the error because Dr. Anesthesiologist did not chart it. Indeed, it would not have been medically unheard of for Mrs. Smith to have completely recovered during the first few days following her surgery, so that the physicians immediately confessing the error would have been as awkward as it would have been premature if Mrs. Smith recovered.

But around the fourth day following the surgery, when Dr. Neurologist took a series of brain scans that showed Mrs. Smith had sustained global brain damage and not a stroke, one could rule out all of Dr. Surgeon's differential diagnoses. By then, it would seem eminently reasonable for the hospital administration to have communicated to the Smith family that the ventilator error was the most likely reason for Betty Smith's condition. By emphasizing it was not an "exact fact" that the ventilator problem was the cause of Mrs. Smith's injury, Dr. Surgeon was neither morally nor clinically convincing in justifying her reluctance to disclose the error. If healthcare communications could only proceed according to whether the communicators were *absolutely* certain of their knowledge or the nature or meaning of their findings, very few communications (or interventions, for that matter) would ever occur. Rather, we hold health professionals to a *reasonable* degree of certainty about etiology, which seems to have been clearly present and available well before the decision was made to discontinue Mrs. Smith's artificial ventilation. However, both the hospital's risk manager and chief nursing officer later remarked at their depositions that at the time of Mrs. Smith's surgery, the hospital had no formal, written policy that addressed disclosure of medical error to patients and families. Apparently, the hospital relied on its personnel who erred to disclose their errors to the harmed parties. And if a physician refused to disclose, then according to the Chief Nursing Officer, "administration should have talked with the physician responsible for the disclosure to get the physician to disclose." If that attempt failed—that is, if the erring physician continued to refuse to disclose the error—it is unclear from the depositions what kind of action the hospital would take to inform the harmed party of error.

As such, it is not surprising that Betty Smith died without her family knowing about this medical error. To the extent that Dr. Anesthesiologist refused to believe and therefore admit that his error was the most likely reason for Mrs. Smith's injury, while the remainder of the treating physicians disowned their responsibility for disclosure, the institution was without a formal mechanism whereby disclosure could occur. Failing Dr. Anesthesiologist's disclosure of the error, it appeared that a "diffusion of responsibility" attitude occurred such that no one felt responsible for the Smith family's ignorance of the ventilator problem. This unfortunately left Dr. Pulmonologist and Dr. Neurologist in the awkward position of managing Patty and Michael Smith's anguish, all the while knowing that information about a crucial aspect of their mother's clinical situation was being withheld from them.

Minimization/Maximization

In light of the unanticipated and tragic dimensions of Betty Smith's outcome, her condition could not be minimized or trivialized by her health professionals. What they did was minimize their moral advocacy for her and her family, as that advocacy involved truth-telling about the ventilator error. But as we will see in the next chapter, that minimization often aggravates the anxiety and anguish of the patient or family members, who then experience the minimization as a dismissal of their concerns and needs. As such, they will likely feel that the trust they explicitly placed in the health professionals is violated, which will make them feel abandoned and betrayed.

One manifestation of the moral minimization of Drs. Surgeon and Anesthesiologist involves their waiting over 50 hours before talking to the Smith family. By itself, that lack of professional contact had an alienating and infuriating effect on Patty and Michael Smith. Michael later said at his deposition:

> It was an early in the morning until late at night deal, hoping we could find a doctor, a health care provider that could give us some kind of idea of what was going on. Because we were beginning to really be suspect, when—when people treat you like you're radioactive material; and it—it was amazing … We need to know what the heck's going on here, and it—it's like it was falling on deaf ears.

Patty remarked:

> We were trying to put together a picture of what had happened best we could. It was—it was like being in the Twilight Zone. It was like—I—I don't know what to tell you other than it was like the day you saw the—the—the airplane go into the World Trade Center … we were trying to put together what—what had happened, what kind of progress we've made; and—we were just trying to get a grip.

When that conversation finally occurred, Dr. Surgeon and Dr. Anesthesiologist minimized or truncated its content by deleting what was clearly the most salient aspect of Mrs. Smith's surgery which, by then, was the leading explanation of her condition. The purposeful deletion of the ventilator problem must have caused Drs. Surgeon and Anesthesiologist tremendous anxiety during that conversation, which one can only think was picked up by Patty and Michael Smith. Patty later said in her deposition:

> I flat didn't trust them … They couldn't tell me what happened to her. I couldn't believe they couldn't tell me what happened to her. I could not believe somebody couldn't tell me when she didn't get air. I just couldn't

believe it. And then Dr. Surgeon stood there and told me I wasn't going to pin it on her. And … my trust just kind of went right out the window right then.

At her deposition, Dr. Surgeon noted the painful effect that withholding information was having on Patty and Michael Smith:

I learned that—that—you know, that you have a family that—that is tremendously distraught over a situation, that you can't entrust other people to communicate with them, that, you know, your responsibility is to make sure that they have the necessary information.

Interestingly, the one health professional who Patty and Michael Smith came to respect and trust was Dr. Neurologist, largely because he spent considerable time with them, was compassionate, and elaborately explained their mother's condition. Indeed, Dr. Neurologist's categorical elimination of stroke from the list of potential causes of Betty Smith's brain injury only reinforced Patty and Michael Smith's suspicion that they were not being told all the facts of their mother's case. Michael remembered Dr. Neurologist as

…extremely helpful. He was talkative. I mean, he—he sat and took time as opposed to a rushed hallway conversation. He sat with us. He—he let us ask questions. He tried to explain it to us. We felt—I at least felt a little bit of comfort that—that at least we felt like somebody was on our side.

Yet, even Dr. Neurologist contained his moral advocacy for the Smiths within the compass of his consultation role. He used the fact that Dr. Anesthesiologist did not chart the ventilator problem to justify his own ignorance of what really happened, and he refused to return Dr. Anesthesiologist's phone call and thus possibly learn more. He referred the ventilator error to administration less than a day after learning of it, but did not follow up to see if the family was ever informed of the error.

Nevertheless, of the various physicians involved in this case, Dr. Neurologist probably went farthest to comfort and ethically advocate for the Smiths. He pursued neurological testing of Mrs. Smith to confirm the diagnosis and rule out stroke; he recommended an autopsy; he told the unvarnished truth to Patty and Michael Smith about their mother's neurological status and comforted and supported them as they decided on discontinuing their mother's artificial ventilation. Also, and perhaps most telling, he remarked in his deposition that he "told the family … that something terrible had happened, in the operating room presumably, and I wasn't there, and so they needed to perform a complete investigation." Ironically, Dr. Neurologist's ethical sensibilities present a case in point to any healthcare team that is cognizant about a harm-causing medical error but resists its disclosure. The fact is, very frequently at least one member of the team might be troubled about concealment and might in various ways, hint, suggest, or imply to the harmed parties that something is dreadfully awry—an implication that might only, as seen in this case, reinforce what those parties already suspect.

For Patty and Michael Smith, the 10 days their mother spent in the hospital were indescribably agonizing. Theirs was an unremitting experience of grief, emotional pain, and bewilderment:

> *Patty:* I never saw her open her eyes except for once. She opened her eyes one time, and it was awful. She looked like a person who somebody had just beat the fool out of. That was the look in her eye. And I felt like oh, my God. She's in there just thinking why won't you help me out of here. That's the feeling I got, just whipped; like somebody had just whipped her to a pulp ... And I decided oh, my gosh, this is horrible what I'm doing here, letting her lay in here like this ...

> *Attorney:* Now, you've indicated that had you known the information (i.e., about the ventilator problem), you probably would have made a decision to discontinue life-support sooner?

> *Patty:* Oh, yes. I think it would have made a very big difference. Frankly, I wish I'd have done it the first day ... [S]he would just be beside herself that we were letting her lay there like that. I mean, if I'm laying there, I'm just begging for somebody to come help me; and I didn't help her. I couldn't help her. I certainly couldn't help her quick enough.

Patty's remark recalls section 8.12 of the AMA Code of Ethics on error disclosure in that withholding significant information from harmed patients or their surrogates deprives those parties of their right to participate in medical decisions. What was perhaps especially anguishing to the Smith family was to realize, months after their mother's death, that they consented to the discontinuation of artificial ventilation without ever knowing the most likely reason for her brain injury. Michael Smith said in his deposition:

> It—it struck me as odd that there was nobody to coordinate the (communication) activity. There's just—there's just people coming and going. There's patients. There's nurses. There's doctors. And we're—we're literally kind of standing in the hallway waiting to see a doctor that we can recognize to try to get some information. So it was highly, highly frustrating. I mean, you can't imagine when your mother's laying around, thrashing around, you don't know what's going to happen. The worst thought in your mind is she's going to be in a comatose state indefinitely ... So finally when we talked to Doctor Neurologist we kind of felt like we had somebody that was taking an interest; because quite frankly, that was my overall impression, that nobody had an interest. This—this is unbelievable. My mother is laying in here in a coma, and nobody has any interest in talking—it was like we were radioactive.

We will let Dr. Surgeon bring this section to a close. At the very end of her deposition, she remarked, "I think that I learned a lesson," which was:

I think I learned the lesson that communication skills—better communications skills should be—that when something really bad happens like this, that from my standpoint, communication skills should be better exercised … I learned that perhaps that—you know, from my own standpoint, that I should try and be more aggressive about a diagnosis and not just about management.

Dr. Surgeon's remark recalls how the fixated-on-treatment narcissist of Chapter 3 can react. The management of thorny moral issues can be easily dismissed in favor of what fixated-on-treatment persons find much more comfortable: managing the treatment plan. As Dr. Surgeon learned, however, this case shows how that treatment-oriented inclination can be interpreted by patients and their families as an act of moral abandonment.

Medical Narcissism

This case vividly illustrates the way medical narcissism differs from its more pathological manifestations. For example, the depositions do not present any allegations by the Smiths of grandiose, arrogant, or imperious behavior from any of the physicians. Moreover, there is no noticeable emotional exploitation on the physicians' parts, short of Patty Smith's alleging deception in the conversation she and her brother had on Wednesday night with Drs. Surgeon and Anesthesiologist. Furthermore, the Smiths particularly emphasized Dr. Neurologist's caring and compassionate behavior, which in his own deposition, Dr. Neurologist called attention to as therapeutically important.

Rather, the narcissistic moments peculiar to this case and not unfamiliar, probably in many cases like it, are represented by the injury or assault that an error coupled with a tragic outcome presents to the healthcare professional's psyche; the fact that such an event horrifically denies whatever expectation of narcissistic reward the healthcare professional usually experiences; the subsequent unavailability or emotional distance effected by the professionals most wounded by the incident; and the way the medical narcissist predictably does the only things he or she knows how to do in such situations: immerse him- or herself in the clinical rather than in the other-regarding dimensions of the case and concoct a brace of explanations and rationalizations that justify this self-protective distancing.

Calling upon exactly the kind of moral inattentiveness that Goleman's model described in Chapter 2, the professionals in this case chose to focus on the clinical details of the case as a proxy for their moral obligation to effect a discussion of the error with Dr. Anesthesiologist and the harmed parties. Having to face the reality of what transpired or any aspects of the error is so frightening or distasteful that Dr. Neurologist even refuses to speak to Dr. Anesthesiologist, claiming that to do so will only distract him from his clinical obligations to the Smiths.

The medical narcissist will predictably take cover and not get any nearer to an error than he or she has to because of his or her immense need to protect his or her vulnerability. Thus, we see:

- Dr. Surgeon's attempt to convince perhaps herself as well as the Smiths that their mother's neurological event was due to "stroke";
- Drs. Surgeon's and Anesthesiologist's conscious and probably unconscious attempt to control the content of the Smith's understanding of what happened (e.g., Dr. Surgeon's numerous etiologic hypotheses; her "stroke" euphemism; the alleged lie in Drs. Surgeon's and Anesthesiologist's confession of ignorance as to how Mrs. Smith could have stopped breathing);
- Dr. Surgeon underlining the fact to the Smiths, on apparently at least two occasions, that Mrs. Smith's adversity involved an anesthesiologic and not surgical event;
- No one having the moral courage to sit down with the Smiths at any time to discuss the ventilator error although Drs. Neurologist and Pulmonologist wasted little time informing hospital administration—perhaps in compliance with the hospital's sentinel event policy, but also perhaps to make sure that administration knew where to place the blame;
- A complicity among Drs. Surgeon, Neurologist, and Pulmonologist to protect one of their own by failing to effect a disclosure of the error to the Smiths;
- A refusal among the physicians, save for Dr. Neurologist, to empathize with the Smiths' agony of incomprehension and to acknowledge their need for truthful disclosure;
- Dr. Anesthesiologist, years after the event, continuing to maintain an unreasonable denial of the most likely cause of Mrs. Smith's injury and refusing to answer the Smith's lawyer's question as to whether or not the ventilator error failed to accommodate the standard of care;
- All the physicians explaining their failure to effect error disclosure by arguing that their duty consisted only in the clinical management of Mrs. Smith's care; and
- No one calling attention to the systemic nature of the error, that is, the mechanical failure of the bed, the X-ray cassette slot malfunction, and the disabled monitoring equipment, perhaps because each individual was singularly attentive to protecting his or her welfare.

The end result of all these behaviors is the Smiths' impression of psychological and moral disengagement. As Michael Smith said, "Nobody had an interest." True to form, when the medical narcissist is confronted with the possibility of a serious harm-causing error, his or her management of it will likely result in an empathic disaster.

A Final Point on Systemic Error

This chapter focused on the way the anxieties and emotional discomforts of the treating professionals affected their moral advocacy for their patient and the patient's family. I would be remiss not to point out, though, that this case also corroborates the systemic theory of harm-causing medical error.

Recall that Dr. Anesthesiologist, upon turning off the ventilator, was disturbed by the failure of the operating table's gear to lower Mrs. Smith as well as by the X-ray cassette that was stuck in its slot. At that moment, Dr. Anesthesiologist claimed he thought he turned the ventilator back to the "on" position and then got up to assist. When he returned to his station, however, he was unaware, or so he claimed, that the various alarms that usually go off when a patient's oxygen level falls to a dangerous point had been programmed to a "suspend indefinite" mode or that their volume was lowered such that they might have been inaudible. Dr. Anesthesiologist claimed he was unaware of the suspend indefinite programming, implying that this was done by and thus with the knowledge of the organization. So, had Dr. Anesthesiologist not left his station because of malfunctioning equipment, had the alarms been properly programmed or audible, and had the surgeon, scrub nurse, or circulating nurse just happened to notice that Mrs. Smith's ventilator was off sooner than Dr. Anesthesiologist, Mrs. Smith's brain injury and its ensuing tragedy might never have occurred. Like so many others, this case is a classic example of system failures coalescing in a way that resulted in a catastrophic outcome.

Chapter 5

Forgiveness

"What is annulled in the act of forgiveness is not the crime itself but the distorting effect that this wrong has upon one's relations with the wrongdoer and perhaps with others." [1, p.17]

Joanna North

Introduction

This chapter will explore various dimensions of forgiveness and especially focus on its unfamiliarity in healthcare. Beginning with psychological and moral characterizations of forgiveness, I will then discuss barriers to the professional's request for forgiveness, the phenomenological trajectory of being wronged, and locating forgiveness within a model of justice. Various ethical as well as psychological arguments that encourage forgiveness will be discussed as well as how narcissistic formations among both victims and offenders frustrate the good that forgiveness can accomplish.

Two Characterizations of Forgiveness

No consensual definition of forgiveness exists.[2] The literature instead offers psychological and moral accounts of forgiveness with two characterizations appearing most prominently.

Psychological characterizations of forgiveness stress its functional aspects as they relate to the present and future psychological health of both victims and offenders. Typically, forgiveness is represented as an act that allows the forgiver to escape or halt repetitive and escalating cycles of resentment and revenge, while it simultaneously allows the forgiven an opportunity to move beyond the transgression and make a new start.[3] One might characterize the forgiver and forgiven phenomenologies with a cognitive-emotive-behavioral triad:[4]

FORGIVENESS FOR THE FORGIVER

Cognitive: "I will stop thinking about the offense."

Emotive: "I will cease to feel anger and hatred toward the offender."

Behavioral: "I will not seek revenge."

FORGIVENESS FOR THE FORGIVEN

Cognitive: "I will acknowledge and admit my wrongdoing."

Emotive: "I will feel and express sorrow for what I did."

Behavioral: "I will desist from committing that wrong again and make amends."

Moral characterizations of forgiveness borrow heavily from the theological literature and presuppose a wrongdoing that normally merits punishment or retribution.[5] A typical justice account depicts the wrongdoer as one who incurs a *moral debt* because he or she violated some justice norm that prescribes what the other is rightfully owed. As such, a number of philosophers, with Kant as the most prominent, repudiated forgiveness as a moral response to wrongdoing since, for them, the only way to right the offense is for the offender to make some kind of calculated reparation to the victim.[6] For these philosophers, there is no moral room for forgiveness, because justice demands that the moral debt be repaid.

The moral context of forgiveness therefore understands it as a supererogatory relinquishment of debt.[7] Forgiveness is supererogatory in that the victim has a legitimate right to recall the debt but forgoes that opportunity. The psychological connotations of forgiveness intersect with the moral ones by characterizing forgiveness as "a willingness to abandon one's right to resentment, negative judgment, and indifferent behavior toward one who unjustly injured us, while fostering the undeserved qualities of compassion, generosity, and even love toward him or her." [8, pp. 46–47]

Although both the psychological and moral accounts of forgiveness will inform the following discussion, it would be well to pay special attention to the latter as it recalls certain arguments from Chapter 2 that dealt with the contractual nature of the health professional-patient relationship. In that chapter I suggested that a harm-causing error counts as a breach of this implicit contract because health professionals hold themselves out to the public as individuals who ply their trade according to professional norms and standards. Thus, if error is defined as an act or judgment that falls below the professional standard, then the professional who commits a harm-causing error has, by definition, breached his or her promise to the client. Consequently, the commission of a harm-causing error not only harms, but it also *wrongs*. The patient suffered an *injustice* that the offender now has a moral duty to rectify. As we will now discuss, positing forgiveness within the moral space of "wronging" facilitates an understanding as to why forgiveness is an alien construct in healthcare environments and why the health professional's requesting the harmed party's forgiveness for a harm-causing error is probably a rare occurrence.

Requesting Forgiveness from the Harmed Party

Although health professionals frequently say "I'm sorry" to patients and families, their declarations are usually meant as expressions of sympathy or compassion rather than genuine requests for forgiveness. The genuine request for forgiveness is not simply a declaration of sorrow but says, in effect, "The wrong you experienced ought not have happened. I am immensely sorry that it did. I ask that you forgive me—that is, that you give up your feelings of anger and revenge and show mercy toward me." [9] Let us examine some reasons why such a supplication by a health professional to a patient is probably a rare occurrence.

The first reason is straightforward. Health professionals should not have a keen familiarity with requesting forgiveness because these requests presuppose that a patient has been wronged, which ought never happen. By definition, licensed health professionals must not deliver care in a way that fails to meet the professional standard, that is, errantly or substandardly. Alternatively, while all clinicians at times witness patients who have poor outcomes, no need to request authentic forgiveness exists when those adverse outcomes are not attributable to substandard care. [10] The health professional who practices entirely within the scope of "reasonableness and prudence" never has to request forgiveness except as a proxy for some other professional who failed to do so. Because serious, harm-causing events that are categorically attributable to error are fairly rare, the request for forgiveness should itself be rare—and therefore unfamiliar to most health professionals.

In addition to the fear of litigation, however, the most likely reasons why professionals resist requesting forgiveness are psychological. If, as Glen Gabbard opined, compulsiveness is a dominant element in the physician's psyche, then these professionals might feel considerable guilt or shame over the commission of an error and perhaps feel that they are not worthy of forgiveness. [11] These individuals may have been (wrongly) taught that the commission of an error is an indication of bad character, about which they should feel ashamed. These intensely painful feelings can compromise the motivation that is required in requesting forgiveness, as they will depress the individual's appreciation of the therapeutic power of forgiveness by arousing his or her feelings of inadequacy and worthlessness.

Alternatively, as the narcissism of certain health professionals encourages their feelings of specialness and superiority, they might feel that they are above asking for forgiveness. [12] They might not feel a need for absolution from the harmed party but, rather, and as we saw in a previous chapter, absolution from their peers. But that only reinforces the narcissistic insularity of the profession and its belief that accountability toward the very persons who place their welfare in the professional's hands is morally unnecessary. The refusal to be accountable to the harmed party tokens either a narcissistic conceit or a complementary, narcissistically based defensiveness that derives from an assault on one's sense of adequacy or competence. As we will examine later on, *even more than confessing error and offering an apology, the request for authentic forgiveness requires a concerted suspension of one's narcissism.* [13]

Ultimately, health professionals are not familiar with requesting compassion and benevolence from patients because doing so implies a profound role reversal. After all, patients are typically the ones who are in need of the professional's power and skill. But to request forgiveness, the professional supplicates him- or herself before the patient and acknowledges the patient's power. And that must seem very odd to the health professional who, day in and day out, is used to bringing his or her expertise to patients who are needy, vulnerable, and disempowered.

PROFESSIONALS REQUESTING FORGIVENESS FROM ONE ANOTHER

While a health professional or healthcare organization has no moral authority to forgive an erring professional for the harm his error caused to the patient—only the harmed party can do that—there are at least two senses in which the erring health professional has incurred a debt to his institution or his peers. The first has already been mentioned: Upon acceptance of employment and then holding themselves out to prospective patient-clients as licensed health professionals, health providers make a public promise that they will practice according to the professional standard of care. Because the commission of a harm-causing error is a serious breach of that public promise, it stands as an example of wronging patient-clients and thus triggers the assumption of a moral debt incurred by the wrongdoer. But notice that the erring professional not only breached his promise to the harmed patient, but also to the institution that hired him, because the employment contract surely proceeded with the explicit understanding that the professional will practice according to the level of competence represented by his licensure or certification. The professional's error violated that organizationally significant expectation and so tokens a moral indebtedness of the employee to the institution. This indebtedness takes on a second and much more concrete meaning when we consider that a professional's error exposes his or her group or institution to legal liability. This is especially pressing if the group or hospital is self-insured because a harm-causing error that results in a malpractice action puts the organization's loss reserves at risk. Since the error might endanger the organization's financial capacity, which is obviously important for the organization's and its employees' welfare, the erring professional incurred an additional debt, now to his or her employer.

A substantial anecdotal history shows, however, that health professionals and their employer organizations have not particularly embraced forgiveness as a customary response to harm-causing error, and only recently—which will be discussed at length in the next chapter—are organizations considering the implementation of a "blameless and nonpunitive" environment for managing their relationship with erring individuals. Rather than forgiveness, organizations have typically ignored or overlooked errors, covered up for or protected an erring professional, or engaged in what is perhaps the most familiar response to error from hospital administration, especially toward non-physician staff members: censure or dismissal.

While a hospital administration's customary blame-and-penalize reaction to error, especially directed toward the non-physician staff, tokens the inequities with which blame and punishment are meted out, one might also hold that blame and punishment manifest a general fear that recommendations of mercy, compassion, empathy, or forgiveness might encourage more errors. Professionals might feel that a policy of forgiveness results in a relaxation of the normal rigor necessary to ensure that errors do not occur. To an even mildly compulsive individual, any prospect that appears to condone or facilitate carelessness or indifference is intolerable.[14]

Indeed, when health professionals are sued for their errors, they experience another unforgiving response, this time anchored in the courts, wherein they face the possibility of having to make some form of financial restitution to the harmed party. If social and cultural factors that surround the commission of errors in American healthcare discourage a health professional's sense of forgiveness, it is not astonishing that professionals do not extend forgiveness to one another or think to ask for it when errors happen.

Even so, my claim that forgiveness—especially as understood within the model of moral indebtedness I am offering—is an unusual response among health professionals seems to contradict Charles Bosk's venerable work on the culture of surgeons, *Forgive and Remember: Managing Medical Failure.*[15] This book resulted from Bosk's doctoral research, in which he gained an intimate familiarity with the surgical department of a teaching hospital in the mid 1970s, and was allowed to observe and record how the training of resident surgeons, whom he called "subordinates," proceeded.

When one reads this book with a view toward the kind of "forgiveness" that was operative among surgeons and their residents, a number of interesting as well as disturbing points emerge. First of all, Bosk differentiates forgivable/punishable errors into two broad categories: technical and normative (or moral). Whereas contemporary research on medical error is largely interested in technical errors—that is, errors of technique, judgment, or system operations—Bosk reported that these kinds of errors were almost reflexively dismissed or forgiven among the "superordinate" or attending surgical staff because everybody made them. Concern over these kinds of errors only becomes prominent when a resident makes them repeatedly or shows a pattern of committing a certain kind of technical error. Indeed, when technical error becomes an object of professional discussion at a morbidity and mortality conference, Bosk describes how the resident's attending physician invariably steps in for the subordinate and takes the blame for not training or supervising the resident carefully enough and thus for "allowing" the error to occur.[16]

The much more serious error, for which decisions about punishment or forgiveness almost certainly arise, is the normative or moral error. Bosk describes these kinds of errors as:

> An individual's failure to acknowledge the underling status which the requirement of "good faith" imposes. The failure to route problems properly because of professional pride or the failure to confess error and admit

shortcomings ... When he makes a moral error, the subordinate shows by his conduct that he does not acknowledge his subordination to the group and its standards ... Just as the group can afford to be merciful in the face of technical error since an individual is contrite, submits himself to group authority, and pledges to do better, the group must be merciless in the face of moral error since an individual is prideful, contemptuous of the group's authority, and offers no assurance of future improvement.[17, p. 180]

A prominent kind of normative error occurs when a resident fails to update an attending physician on an important development in a patient's care or condition. Here, the attending wants to avert "surprises" because "[a] surprise for the attending carries with it the implication that a house staff member was lazy, negligent, or dishonest [while a] normative error in turn carries with it the implication that a fundamental breach of etiquette governing the role relation between doctor and patient has occurred."[18, pp. 53 and 55]

Now, it absolutely must be admitted that the norms that govern the understanding and seriousness of normative error are ultimately grounded in the surgeon's comprehension of his or her duty toward the patient and in insuring that the patient receives optimal care. Nevertheless, there is a remarkable dimension of narcissism in the above characterization of moral error—a narcissism that is not only embedded in the error's affront to the authority status of the attendings, but also evident by the fact that punishment for moral error goes in only one direction: from the top down. Although an attending/superordinate physician might commit a normative error—say, he or she failed to call for an expert consultation that might have prevented a patient's demise—the attending will rarely be severely criticized and virtually never punished. The reasons Bosk offers are that attending surgeons have the privilege of rank and "are directly accountable to no one on a daily basis."[19, p. 58] Their faculty appointments, research publications, and professional awards "are a presumptive moral licensing ... Basically, an attending is not publicly blamed for normative errors because there is no one to accuse him of such moral lapses. No one stands above him in the hierarchy."[20, p. 58] Furthermore, attendings customarily spend much more time lecturing, doing research, and attending to administrative work and so are not as encumbered by the pressures of patient care and their associated opportunities to commit errors. Bosk concludes that, "Rank, moral authority, and everyday task-structure insulate the attending and expose the housestaff to the danger of normative error."[21, p. 58] Attendings never find moral fault with one another, and their subordinates are never allowed to criticize them. "Forgiveness" for moral failure occurs only when the attending decides that the subordinate evinced an acceptable degree of contrition, expansively acknowledged the authority of his supervisors, and redoubled his diligence and efforts to accommodate the needs and expectations of those in power.

In Bosk's account, criticism, error admission, and forgiveness presumably occur at morbidity and mortality conferences, yet even here an odd form of forgiveness reigns. Typically, attendings take the full brunt of criticism for errors although the nature of the criticism that Bosk describes is not so much directed at the attending physician, but rather takes the form of the attending's self-criticism. While a true confessional, the morbidity and mortality conference that Bosk describes is as much a ritualistic ceremony wherein individuals are automatically forgiven just by virtue of their public self-denunciation: "The major punishment of the practice is the embarrassment of a public confessional and the pain the outcome itself actually causes the surgeon's conscience." [22, p. 145] Because going through the paces of the confessional results in almost automatic absolution, Bosk concludes that "this is a hair shirt on the outside only; for the wearer it has the silken lining of unconditional professional support." [23, p. 145]

The model of forgiveness that Bosk describes is odd indeed. It rests upon an insistence that the superiority of the power structure is categorically and unwaveringly affirmed. It describes a right of passage whereby a professional initially proceeds from a position of abject humility that borders on worthlessness to eventually achieving a status of unimpeachable moral standing and grandiosity. Most remarkably, at no time does this model of forgiveness understand the patient—for whom, after all, all of this expertise and training exists—to have any voice in meting out punishment and forgiveness. Rather this model of forgiveness is overwhelmingly insular and accountable only to itself. It and it alone decides which acts are blamable, forgivable, and punishable.

Only recently has that insularity become a matter of public consternation. Certainly, the movement to disclose errors and offer an apology to harmed patients marks a considerable step beyond what Bosk observed 30 years ago. But as the following will show, healthcare organizations still have some way to go to implement a forgiveness construct in their error disclosure practices.

The Significance of Forgiveness

Magdalena Santillan, the mother of Jesica Santillan who was given organs whose blood type was incompatible with hers, said that she wanted Jesica's surgeon to lose his license. When Jesica died and Mrs. Santillan was asked to consider donating Jesica's organs, she reportedly said, "You murdered Jesica … Why would we give you organs to murder other people? " [24, p. 68]

In May 2002, Linda McDougal was told she had breast cancer and she elected to have a double mastectomy. Two days after the operation, it was discovered that Mrs. McDougal's breast biopsy specimen and its related paperwork got mixed up with another patient's records and that Mrs. McDougal did not have cancer. Although she was immediately told of the mistake and received an apology from her surgeon, Mrs. McDougal claimed she did not receive an apology from the pathologist who appeared primarily responsible for the error and was upset that the pathologist was not disciplined: "I think he's got to be penalized," she is quoted as saying. "He's got to be held accountable, and right now they haven't even slapped his wrist." [25, p. 2]

Josie King was 18 months old when she was admitted to Johns Hopkins in January 2001 after she suffered first and second degree burns by climbing into a hot bath. Her mother alleged that Josie died from severe dehydration and inept narcotization. About a year and a half after Josie's death, the hospital created the Josie King Patient Safety Program. Describing her feelings in the wake of Josie's death to a professional audience in Boston, her mother said, "There were days when all I wanted was to destroy the hospital and then put an end to my own pain. My three remaining children were my only reason for getting out of bed and functioning." [26, p. 2]

Dan Wingerd was an investment counselor who received a kidney transplant on the wrong side. He was quoted as saying, "Had this surgery been successful, I would have resumed my career as an investment adviser. I was traveling, which I can't do now; three days a week I'm in dialysis for five hours. I'm getting ready to volunteer at the local district attorney's office to help clear cold cases. It's just to make do to keep from going nuts." [27, p. 2]

It is difficult not to think that reactions such these are fairly typical "victim" responses to catastrophic harm-causing error. As we saw in Chapter 2, the human organism is neurologically wired for self-preservation. The ancient structures of our brains primarily focus on the preservation of our bio-physiological integrity. Whereas philosophers, especially starting with Descartes, contemplate the "solipsistic" nature of consciousness—that is, the fact that I am intractably encased in my sensorium and cannot climb outside it to experience the way others perceive the world or the way the world is "in itself"—psychologists offer this solipsism as an explanation for why I perceive or "feel" myself in a more elaborate and intense fashion than I perceive other selves. [28, p. 93] My intense feeling of myself, especially in instances of serious threat or stress, is an evolutionary derivative of my hard-wired interest in self-preservation. The species that cannot summon a palpable feeling of self-centeredness and self-reference when it is confronted by a predator cannot survive. Consequently, when I or my loved ones—who, after all, are the biological transports of my genetic legacy—are injured or imperiled, feelings of shock, rage, horror, and revenge are natural expressions of my self-preservative interests. Moreover, our feelings of rage toward the perpetrators of harm-causing medical error can be magnified by the realization that the harm perpetrators are the very persons to whom we entrusted our welfare. Our feelings of immense anger will therefore often be punctuated by additional feelings of disbelief and injustice, as in "this shouldn't have happened to me." [29]

Indeed, given the ways our neurological architecture is so bent on maintaining self-regulation and how its stress, fear, and aggression components are deployed to maximize the organism's survival probability, one wonders how forgiveness could have even appeared on our evolutionary landscape. For example, some studies suggest that individuals who retaliate when wronged tend to be wronged less frequently, which only makes forgiveness more problematic and less intuitive. [30]

Newberg and his colleagues noted, however, that progressively escalating revenge can be socially disruptive: "[R]evenge behavior is poorly modulated and can easily lapse into an excessive mutual retaliation owing to an excessive evaluation of the self, with the consequent miscalculation of what is needed to restore equilibrium." [31, p. 99] Perhaps, then, forgiveness, like justice, might be evolutionarily explained as a facilitator in containing vengeful behaviors that can destroy communities. If justice is "the sociocultural attempt to correct the imperfect revenge behavior,"[32, p. 100] forgiveness provides complementary assistance in restoring psychosocial equilibrium so that a wrongful injury is absorbed into an individual's or society's memory in a way that no longer precipitates disturbance or disruption.[33]

Alternatively, the absence of a forgiving response increases the likelihood that the victim's feelings can spiral into increasing bitterness and rage. The harmed individual will be inclined to perceive the offender as someone who is dangerous.[34] If that perception is not changed, the victim may well entertain revenge fantasies. We might especially note the not uncommon reaction among victims to have the oppressor "expelled" from his or her profession by having his or her license revoked. Motivated by a combined desire to punish as well as prevent the offender from committing the wrong again, expulsion of the wrongdoer from his or her community has assumed a variety of forms throughout history such as exile, imprisonment or, in its most severe form, execution.[35]

Because the American legal system allows complainants recourse through the courts, it is hardly surprising that a desire to punish the erring health professional strongly figures as a motive in litigation. That motivation can be understood as an expression of the victim's identity as "having-been-wronged."[36] While a malpractice suit might not change the "been wronged" self-understanding of the victim, it might nevertheless diminish that person's vengeful feelings. Consequently, a goal of the professional who discloses a harm-causing medical error, whether motivated by the desire to avert a malpractice suit or just to help the victim overcome painful feelings of bitterness and rage, ought to aim at defusing the harmed party's emotional pain and his or her construal of the harm-causing error as intentional or as perpetrated by uncaring or inept health professionals.[37]

Even if the victim is not approached by the offender, it is interesting to note that the victim may ultimately forgive the offender because the victim can no longer tolerate his or her intense feelings of bitterness. While forgiveness might be supererogatory, it can also be self-interested. Some victims primarily forgive in order to feel better, only to find out later that their forgiveness has positively affected the offender as well.[38]

Narcissistic Barriers to Requesting or Bestowing Forgiveness

One of the psychological findings on forgiveness is termed the "magnitude gap." Roy Baumeister and his colleagues noted that perpetrators tended to resort to "minimizing interpretations" of the gravity of their transgression or their role in the wrongdoing, while victims tended to perseverate and magnify the severity of the wrong or the wrong-doer.[39] As we have seen, persons harmed by medical error will call for the license of the involved professional to be revoked, despite the fact that he or she may have had an exemplary record up to that time and might not even have been primarily responsible for the wrong. On the other hand and as we saw in Chapter 2, perpetrators will often resort to a host of strategies or ploys to convince themselves that either an error did not occur, or the harm was not serious, or someone else was to blame. Consequently, while the harmed party might be seething with an ever-consuming rage at what happened, the wrongdoer might simultaneously be consoling him- or herself with self-serving distortions or confabulations of the event that relieve him or her of the discomfort of admitting error, apologizing, and seeking forgiveness.[40] This must count as one of the principal reasons why health professionals avoid or excuse themselves from error disclosure conversations, only to become bewildered and then angered over how their unwittingly dismissive behavior prompted the patient's rage and the initiation of a malpractice claim.

Narcissism is a central theme of this book, and it is worthwhile to note how it affects both the victim and the perpetrator of medical error, and by extension diminishes the likelihood of either party's arrival at forgiveness behavior. The error victim's narcissism begins with the neuro-biologically mediated shock and outrage over the injury. Without forgiveness, his or her subsequent reactions can easily evolve into hatred, rage, and revenge.[41] Psychologists note how levels of narcissism are inversely related to forgiving behavior, and therefore how narcissists may be "forgiveness challenged." Robert Emmons noted how forgiveness:

> Requires a humbling of the self and a relinquishment (at least temporarily) of grandiosity. Forgiveness also requires abandoning the egocentric position of seeing others in light of one's own needs and developing insights into the offender's own motives, needs, and reasons for acting as he or she did. In other words, the person takes a more empathic view of the other's behavior. The third and final step of the forgiveness process involves a commitment not to engage in "retributive opportunities" (i.e., taking vengeance). All three of these steps may be close to insurmountable tasks for narcissistic individuals.[42, p. 166]

The narcissistic transgressor, on the other hand, is likely to resist acknowledging his guilt and thus unlikely to offer an apology, not to mention request forgiveness. Because of the narcissist's desire to maintain his or her fantasy of perfection, he or she may be unable to admit fault. In considering the narcissist's idea of an apology, Emmons observed that it never loses its self-referentiality, that is, "I can't believe that I did that," or "You must think I'm a terrible person," or "I don't blame you if you never forgive me."[43, p. 167] While these may seem attempts at apology, Emmons suggested that they really aim to evoke reassurance from the victim that despite the transgression, the transgressor is, at bottom, perfect.[44]

Last, a shame versus a guilt reaction might influence the extent to which one requests forgiveness. Whereas guilt is often associated with an action or event that merits some kind of reparation, shame connotes a feeling of self-loathing wherein the shamed individual wants to hide.[45] Exline and Baumeister observed that shame-prone offenders are more susceptible to anger, suspiciousness, blame shifting, and aggressive behavior than guilt-prone individuals.[46] So, while feelings of guilt might incline an offender to seek absolution, feelings of shame might prompt him or her to withdraw, hide the offense, and deflect or simply deny responsibility. Consequently, to the extent that health providers are taught that the commission of medical error tokens a serious character flaw rather than a system failure, their inclination to conceal error becomes understandable (although not justifiable) as a shame response. The tremendous desire of an ashamed individual to save face can simply overwhelm whatever inclination toward public repentance he might otherwise have.

As with oppressors, so with victims: When the latter have a similarly strong desire to save face or when they are ashamed of being victimized by error, they might resort to revenge. While the best remedy would be to find some mechanism that restores these individuals' sense of power and wholeness, victims of error who have an especially vulnerable, easily humiliated, easily assaulted sense of self are less likely to forgive. Commentators point out that either for the victim or the transgressor, forgiveness begins with a humbling of the self. As such, the narcissist is forgiveness challenged.[47]

The Trajectory of Forgiveness

Let us recall Mr. Thompson's case as described in the Chapter 2. Mr. Thompson received 100 units of insulin when he was supposed to receive 10 units. He progressed into insulin shock and required resuscitation and transfer to intensive care. Although he recovered fully despite the error, his physician tried very hard to withhold acknowledgment of the error and, in so doing, was acutely unempathic to Mr. Thompson, whose anger only escalated with each question he asked. Suppose Mr. Thompson's physician, instead of hedging and obfuscating as to what happened, told Mr. Thompson of the error and then said:

> Mr. Thompson, this should not have happened, and we are sorry beyond words. There was nothing that you did to make this happen. It was something we did and it was entirely our fault. I can't imagine how upset you might be over this, and you have a perfect right to feel angry. For all of us, Mr. Thompson, I am so sorry that this happened and that you suffered so needlessly. Please forgive us.

What effect might this declaration have had on both Mr. Thompson and his physician?

First, consider that a harm-causing error such as the one Mr. Thompson experienced creates a moral breach in the professional-patient relationship because the patient was frankly wronged. The plea for forgiveness is thus a first attempt to mend that breach. It is an attempt to restore trust and to repair a relationship that has been marred by an unfortunate and unjustifiable incident.[48]

Now, while this might serve as an abstract formulation of forgiveness, it does not describe Mr. Thompson's psychological reaction to the plea for forgiveness. More probably than not, his experience of the physician's apology and plea for forgiveness will at least be that his suffering from the error *is being honored.*[49] In the original scenario, this honoring is precisely what did not happen and explains why Mr. Thompson's ire increased with his every question. What the physician's apology and forgiveness declaration would accomplish is confirmation of Mr. Thompson's self-understanding as someone who was unjustifiably wronged. By frankly admitting the wrong and emphasizing that Mr. Thompson had nothing to do with it, the physician empathically validates Mr. Thompson's belief that, "I'm a good and decent person who did not deserve for this horrible thing to happen." By telling Mr. Thompson that he has a perfect right to be angry, the physician confirms Mr. Thompson's feelings and thus *contains* them. One of the amazing features of the empathic response consists in how its other-affirmation creates a bond between the parties. By sensing that the physician deeply understands his emotions, the patient finds it all the more difficult to escalate his anger and rage.[50]

Notice, however, that a failure to acknowledge an error, not to mention failing to apologize for it, will be interpreted by the patient who eventually finds it out as, "Well, this error did in fact happen and it harmed me. Obviously, my doctors and nurses did not care enough about me to prevent the error from happening, which was all the more confirmed by their deciding not to tell me what happened. They don't acknowledge their mistakes. They don't apologize for them. They just don't care." Small wonder such patients contemplate lawsuits.

By containing the psychological damage that the error causes, the apology and request for forgiveness annul not the error itself "but the distorting effect that this wrong has upon one's relations with the wrongdoer and perhaps with others."[51, p. 17] Over the years I have received a number of phone calls from persons who believe they have been wronged by health professionals. Two things stand out in such conversations. The first is that the caller repeats everything he or she says to me at least a half dozen times. Persons who feel grievously wronged tend to perseverate on every salient detail of the wrong. Absent the caller's outrage, these calls should last anywhere from 5 to 15 minutes. Instead, some callers could talk for hours. And that reveals the second feature of such calls. The intensity of the caller's feelings makes it seem that his or her life is consumed by what happened.[52] Of course, this would hardly be a surprise if the harm results in disablement, so that the caller is constantly reminded of how his quality of life has been damaged. What is quite sad about listening to such callers, however, is that no matter how grave or modest their injury, their sense of betrayal and outrage is immense, largely from not having received any expression of compassion from the health professional. It is precisely that absence of emotion from the health professional that adds insult to their injury. Tragically, such victims are unable to transcend their injury. Deprived of an apology and an opportunity to forgive, their bitterness becomes all-consuming.

This raises an interesting feature of forgiveness in medical contexts, in that the individual who usually finds him- or herself most changed by forgiveness is the forgiver, not the forgiven.[53] Whereas an apology may soothe the listener, the health professional who requests his or her patient's forgiveness is calling upon the patient's moral sensibilities and asking that a change occur in the patient's interpretation of the wrong. Bestowing forgiveness requires that the victim-patient set aside his or her right to revenge and reframe the wrongdoer-professional as someone capable of doing better.[54] It asks, "Can you relinquish your right to punish me and can you trust me again?" The act of requesting forgiveness encourages the victim to interpret the wrong differently from the way he or she would without an acknowledgment of the error, an apology, and a request for forgiveness. Just as the request for forgiveness reinforces the victim's self-perception as an individual who did not deserve this wrong to happen, so it encourages the victim's perception of the wrongdoer as one who did not mean for the wrong to occur and who is appropriately chastened by it. Forgiveness is an act that seeks to heal the future of the relationship, which only the forgiver can do.[55]

Commentators note that forgiveness can be immensely therapeutic for victims. Enright and North characterized the forgiver as thinking, "If I can do this, forgive him, then I can't have been totally destroyed by his actions. I am something over and above the harm which he has done to me; otherwise I couldn't be offering him forgiveness here and now."[56, p. 19] This is clearly what my telephone callers cannot do. Absent the offender's apology or resorting to the courts, they are deprived of any sort of relief from the wrong they have experienced.

Forgiveness attempts to restore a reciprocated sense of humanity to the ruptured relationship. The forgiveness requester seeks to restore the victim's disrupted identity, while the forgiver acts to restore the wrongdoer's self-respect and self-worth. Indeed, the act of forgiving may well be motivated by an empathic impulse from the victim in that he or she understands that the wrongdoer also has suffered from the wrong. By reframing the wrongdoer, the patient understands the professional as separate from the wrong and as pressured by work demands that were perhaps over and above his control and that facilitated the wrongdoing. Indeed, where the victim forgives without the offender's apology, it may be because the injured party is able to set aside his or her rage and appreciate the wrongdoer's inability to request forgiveness as a result of his or her developmental history.[57]

Justice and Forgiveness

Some philosophers repudiate forgiveness and laud the justice value of resentment. For them, wrongdoers infringe on the moral order so that resentment and its resulting demand for retribution put the moral world back into balance. Theirs is a "philosophical resentment" that looks to the social value of how vengeance, triggered by unjustifiable wronging, restores our sense of self-respect and sends a message to those who would try to dishonor it.[58]

I have been impressed, however, with counterarguments that frame resentment as not a final but an intermediate step in the phenomenology of wronging. While it may be inevitable that most persons' experience of being wronged begins in shock, anger, and resentment, their deciding to take up a long-term psychological residence in a world of pain and bitterness is hardly beneficial or healthy. Indeed, there is some reason to believe that their inability to move forward indicates a narcissistically unhealthy sense of self. Jean Hampton noted that "we resent only those persons who have the power to humiliate us,"[59, p. 53] and we have seen how certain narcissistic types are especially vulnerable to the pain of such embarrassment. When resentment becomes one of the salient nodes of one's existence, life loses much of its joy and positive energy. It is hard to imagine how a victim can benefit from clinging to his or her hatred and outrage.[60] Thus, the health professional who commits error but withholds an acknowledgment, apology, and request for forgiveness from the harmed party deprives him or her of an opportunity to transcend the wrong and the emotional pain connected with the possibility of lingering, perseverative bitterness.

Note, however, that in none of this does the offender ask the victim to forget the wrong-doing. Rather, the victim is asked to recollect the incident with mercy rather than with "grievance-oriented remembering."[61, p. 61] The power of an apology and the act of forgiveness locates the wrong in the past, not the present, and thus makes possible the morally ideal attitude that any two persons, even victim and offender, can have toward one another: respect.

Conclusion

Psychological factors and institutional cultures have long thwarted the appearance of a forgiveness sensibility in healthcare. Yet, the above shows that once the therapeutic value of forgiveness is realized, it can be immensely healing in instances of harm-causing error. Indeed, there is some evidence that if forgiveness halts those feelings of revenge that frequently motivate malpractice suits, it might also serve to contain the revenge behaviors that motivate plaintiffs' seeking huge monetary awards.[62]

Coming to accept the value of forgiveness in instances of harm-causing error will probably require nothing short of a "paradigm change" whereby the attitudes, values, beliefs, and the historically enculturated roles of health professionals and patients are overhauled. The next chapter offers some recommendations toward that end.

References

1. North, Joanna. "The 'ideal' of forgiveness: A philosopher's exploration." In *Exploring Forgiveness*, eds. Robert D. Enright and Joanna North. Madison, WI: The University of Wisconsin Press, 1998, pp. 3–34.

2. McCullough, Michael E.; Pargament, Kenneth I.; and Thoresen, Carl E. "The psychology of forgiveness." In *Forgiveness: Theory, Research, and Practice*, eds. Michael E. McCullough, Kenneth I. Pargament, and Carl E. Thoresen. New York: The Guilford Press, 2000, pp. 1–14.

3. Govier, Trudy. *Forgiveness and Revenge*. London: Routledge, 2002.

4. North, 1998.

5. Exline, Julie Juola, and Baumeister, Roy F. "Expressing forgiveness and repentance." In McCullough, Pargament, and Thoresen, 2000, pp. 133–157.

6. Shriver, Donald W. *An Ethic for Enemies: Forgiveness in Politics*. New York: Oxford University Press, 1995.

7. Enright, Robert D.; Freedman, Suzanne; and Rique, Julio. "The psychology of interpersonal forgiveness." In Enright and North, 1998, pp. 46–62.

8. Enright, Freedman, and Rique, 1998.

9. Shriver, 1995.

10. North, 1998.

11. Exline and Baumeister, 2000.

12. Emmons, Robert A. "Personality and forgiveness." In McCullough, Pargament, and Thoresen, 2000, pp. 156–175.

13. Emmons, 2000.

14. Gabbard, Glen O. "The role of compulsiveness in the normal physician." *JAMA*. 254(20):2926–2929. Also see Bernstein, Albert J. *Emotional Vampires: Dealing with People Who Drain You Dry*. New York: McGraw Hill, 2001.

15. Bosk, Charles. *Forgive and Remember: Managing Medical Failure*. Chicago: The University of Chicago Press, 1979.

16. Bosk, 1979.

17. Bosk, 1979.

18. Bosk, 1979.

19. Bosk, 1979.

20. Bosk, 1979.

21. Bosk, 1979.

22. Bosk, 1979.

23. Bosk, 1979.

24. Comarow, Avery. Jesica's story. *U.S. News & World Report*, July 28/August 4: 51–54, 56, 58, 60, 62, 66, 68, 70, 72, 2003.

25. Howatt, Glenn. Lab's mistake haunts woman as she talks about her loss. Available at http://www.startribune.com. Dated 1/21/2003.

26. Sorrel's speech to IHI Conference, October 11, 2002. Available at http://www.josieking.org. Dated 2/24/2003.

27. Burton, Susan. The biggest mistake of their lives. Available at http://www.nytimes.com. Dated 3/16/2003.

28. Newberg, Andrew; d'Aquili, Eugene G.; Newberg, Stephanie K.; and deMarici, Verushka. "The neuropsychological correlates of forgiveness." In McCullough, Pargament, and Thoresen, 2000, pp. 91–110.

29. Enright, Freedman, and Rique, 1998.

30. Newberg et al., 2000.

31. Newberg et al., 2000.

32. Newberg et al., 2000.

33. Newberg et al., 2000.

34. Newberg et al., 2000.

35. Shriver, 1995.

36. Fitzgibbons, Richard. "Anger and the healing power of forgiveness: A psychiatrist's view." In Enright and North, 1998, pp. 63–74.

37. Fitzgibbons, 1998.

38. Enright, Freedman, and Rique, 1998.

39. Exline and Baumeister, 2000.

40. Govier, 2002.

41. Newberg et al., 2000.

42. Emmons, 2000.

43. Emmons, 2000.

44. Emmons, 2000.

45. Exline and Baumeister, 2000.

46. Exline and Baumeister, 2000.

47. Emmons, 2000.

48. Govier, 2002.

49. Govier, 2002.

50. Govier, 2002.

51. North, 1998.

52. North, 1998.

53. Enright, Freedman, and Rique, 1998.

54. Govier, 2002.

55. Enright, Freedman, and Rique, 1998.

56. North, 1998.

57. Govier, 2002.

58. Enright, Freedman, and Rique, 1998.

59. Govier, 2002.

60. Govier, 2002.

61. Govier, 2002.

62. Govier, 2002.

Chapter 6

Remedies

"Anyone who has ever known doctors well enough to hear medical shop talk, without reserve, knows that they are full of stories about each other's blunders and errors ... But no doctor dare accuse another of malpractice. He is not sure enough of his own [reputation] to ruin another man by it ... I do not blame him; I should do the same myself. But the effect of this state of things is to make the medical profession a conspiracy to hide its own shortcomings."

George Bernard Shaw, *The Doctor's Dilemma, 1902*

Introduction

If health professionals are to disclose error in a morally adequate, patient-centered manner, they need at least three kinds of support. In order of moral importance, the first is surely a structured curriculum along with a brace of learning experiences whereby they might better understand the nature of humanistic medicine and gain insight into how their psychological formations and use of "self" powerfully affect their relationships with patients. Largely, this type of training takes the form of observations of ideal, role-model behaviors, students' practicing these behaviors with iterative critiques of their relational and empathic behaviors, and professionals becoming deeply "mindful" of their personal beliefs, feelings, attitudes, and values. This latter exploration especially involves the professional's reflection on and analysis of his or her reactions to emotionally painful situations such as are aroused by anticipating the disclosure of medical error. The hope is that as these experiences unfold and are absorbed, the health professional's moral formation will incline toward a straightforward and compassionate disclosure of error.

A second source of support is for the professional to find him- or herself in a "moral atmosphere" that encourages ethical behavior and truth telling and that repudiates the avoidance of medical error acknowledgment and concealment. A much discussed element in realizing this kind of moral environment is for the organization to develop a "nonpunitive and blameless" ideology such that health professionals will not have to fear organizational recrimination, censure, and other penalties for acknowledging and reporting unintentional errors. Not only will such environments resist blame or censure, but they also will train staff to counsel and support health professionals in their disclosure of an error to the harmed party.

A third support is tort reform. While health professionals ought to do the right thing regardless of whatever burdens are associated with it, many of them will resist doing so as long as they are convinced that frank and truthful error disclosure will result in a painful and costly malpractice action. Indeed, of these three supports, relieving the health professional from fear of tort litigation or its consequences might have the most favorable effect on improving the rate and quality of error disclosures.

But because I want to examine these supports as they increasingly offer moral, rather than simply practical, remedies toward encouraging error disclosure, I will present them in the reverse order than is offered above. Beginning with the least morally persuasive but perhaps most practical and influential factor that would favorably affect error disclosure, namely, tort reform, I will proceed to discuss how a morally conscientious organization might understand the implementation of a "blameless and nonpunitive" policy to manage error reporting. As we will see, developing such an environment, while laudable, not only presents thorny problems about assessment of responsibility, blame, and punishment, but the blameless and nonpunitive environment is only an intermediate point toward implementing an honest and truthful policy for disclosing medical error.

Consequently, I will end the chapter with a lengthy examination of organizational and curricular strategies that might influence the professional's moral formation in a patient-centered way. The goal of this last section will be to list and discuss a number of variables that might inform and direct a journey of self-exploration and its intersection with empathy such that at its end, a professional discloses error simply because concealment is understood as a non-option.

SECTION 1 ■ TORT REFORM

The Malpractice Crisis

As these lines are being written in late Fall of 2003, physicians in at least half of the United States are reeling from skyrocketing malpractice insurance premiums.[1] A somewhat typical example, reported in late summer 2002 by the *Atlanta Journal Constitution,* is Dr. Jim Luckie from Fitzgerald, Georgia.[2] Dr. Luckie runs a family practice in this south-central Georgia town, population 9,000, and performs about 30 deliveries a year. Although he has never been successfully sued, Dr. Luckie was informed that over the next few years, his malpractice premiums would increase from $12,000 to $28,000 a year. Dr. Luckie's reluctant response was to stop delivering babies in order to contain his insurance costs. The same article reported that Dr. Clay Burnett, a Savannah cardiovascular surgeon, paid $47,000 for malpractice insurance in 2001, but the best quote he was able to find in 2002 was $243,880. Dr. Burnett was quoted as saying, "I'm going to look at all options even if it means moving to another state."[3, p. Q8]

The phenomenon of physicians giving up part of their practice or moving out of state because of excessively high malpractice costs can create a serious public health, and therefore ethical, problem. Many women seeking prenatal or obstetrical care in rural Georgia are hard pressed to find a physician who will care for them and deliver their babies.[4] On the other side of the United States, Nevada physicians have been hit particularly hard with rising malpractice premiums, causing emergency departments to shut down and riveting the attention of the state legislature on reforming the state's tort system.[5] Because the provision of health services is an obvious societal good, government would appear to have a duty to remedy the problem of hospitals or physicians that risk bankruptcy from a huge malpractice award because no commercial insurance was available for them to purchase.

Nevertheless, this book is about the ethical dimensions of medical error. Although one might certainly sympathize with attempts by physicians and hospitals to find affordable premiums, one might also argue that the patient who suffered harm from a health professional's or health organization's error most certainly has a right to recover whatever damages he or she is reasonably owed. Patients do not have a legal duty to assume the harms that might befall them from professional error, so that courts have invalidated the occasional attempts of hospitals to have patients sign waivers upon admission that relieve the institution or its employees from liability in the event of a harm-causing error.[6]

Furthermore, one of the fundamental arguments of this book, which has been endorsed by the American Medical Association since 1981, is that errors should be truthfully and honestly disclosed regardless of their legal consequences.[7] Some readers might therefore argue that from a purely moral point of view, a discussion about the emotional discomfort connected with doing the right thing, such as disclosing error, is out of place in this book, and that the following observations on tort reform—so that health professionals might feel more encouraged to do the right thing—constitute moral crassness. One does the right thing because it is right, not because of any salutary or odious consequences the act engenders.

Specifically, various tort reform measures might include:[8]

- Limits on what plaintiffs might claim by way of noneconomic damages (i.e., over and above lost wages and medical costs that result from the negligence)
- Striking down joint and several liability (i.e., replacing each defendant's liability for 100 percent of the judgment with apportioning damages according to the degree of fault attributed to each defendant)

- More stringent criteria for qualifying expert witnesses
- Limits on punitive damages
- Reducing the plaintiff's award if he or she somehow contributed to the negligence, such as a patient who fails to comply with his or her physician's orders
- Limits on attorney compensation

While these measures might well diminish a health professional's fears over honest disclosure of error because he or she has less to lose from doing so, they have nevertheless received considerable criticism. A key economic criticism leveled at them is that even if they are passed, they will not improve the economic climate for insurance companies and their insureds.[9] For example, a familiar argument among insurers and insureds is that runaway jury verdicts are a primary reason for premium hikes. Others counterargue that the real reason premiums have skyrocketed is that insurers underpriced their premiums during much of the 90s because their stock portfolios were performing outstandingly well. When the market tanked at the end of the decade, insurers had to recover their losses with an explosion in premium increases.[10] Other research suggests that caps on damages do not contain premiums. In 1975, California adopted caps of $250,000 on noneconomic damages, only to see health professional premiums skyrocket for the next decade, reaching an all-time high in 1988.[11]

The moral substance of the tort reform criticism, on the other hand, is that most if not all of these measures ultimately boil down to making it more difficult for plaintiffs to sue and recover damages without any compensating benefit for those patients who suffered from negligent acts. Because tort reform measures are markedly oriented toward the welfare of physicians and healthcare institutions, they present an unambiguous moral threat to preserving the patient's right of redress for whatever wrongs he or she sustained. Caps on noneconomic or punitive damages that are set at $250,000, for example, are said to discriminate against individuals who have been profoundly harmed by negligence and who, by virtue of the cap, are disallowed from recovering what might otherwise compensate for lifelong suffering and misery.[12]

Consider the following example, which is based on a real case: A couple unable to have children opted for in-vitro fertilization. After harvesting several of the woman's eggs and fertilizing them with her husband's sperm, the embryos were implanted in her uterus and three healthy fetuses developed. The couple decided to selectively abort one, but unbeknownst to the physician performing the procedure, the abortion failed and the fetus, although damaged by the abortion attempt, survived. Despite numerous sonograms that apparently failed to detect a third fetal heart beat, three infants were born, one with dreadful anomalies. This child required multiple surgeries during its early years and, even in a best-case scenario, will have significant disability for the entirety of its life. If there was negligence on the physician's part, one wonders if it is enough to only award economic damages to this child and his family, in view of how various aspects of this horror will affect the quality of their lives and their relationships for as long as they live.

We are thus confronted with a dilemma whose terms are discouraging: 1) Change the tort system so that physicians can practice medicine more comfortably and disclose errors more truthfully because they have less to lose—with the consequence that some patients harmed by error will have a lessened opportunity to recover what they are owed; or 2) Leave the system as it is—with the consequences that many patients who suffered harm will sue physicians just to find out what happened, with many of those suits succeeding for plaintiffs such that, at the current rates of premium increases and exodus of insurers from the marketplace, the tort system might eventually capsize.

Is there a third option, however, that not only affords harmed patients a reasonable recovery but is cost-effective among physician-purchasers, and that also reduces the health professional's anxiety over being harshly penalized for error disclosure? Two such legislative remedies have been advanced and touted as able to do just that: enterprise liability and no-fault.

Enterprise Liability

Enterprise liability is an amalgam of various legal forms of liability—notably, vicarious liability, agency, and corporate liability—that essentially make an organization responsible for the wrongs of its workers.[13] Even though no pure system of enterprise liability currently exists in American healthcare, hospitals are commonly included in lawsuits wherein one or more of their employees or independent physician contractors is sued for negligence. Thus, a hospital that employs a number of anesthesiologists as salaried workers will be sued under a long-standing notion known as vicarious liability, wherein the employer is held liable for the wrongs its employees commit while performing job functions. Just so, a private practice physician who employs a nurse or physician assistant is liable for the latter's mistake if it occurs in the performance of the employee's job functions.[14]

Most physicians, however, are self- or group-employed and contract their services out to hospitals. Courts hold, however, that patients usually know nothing about the business relationships between physicians and the hospitals in which they practice. Rather, courts assume that the only thing the patient knows is that the hospital in which he finds himself "provides" or "holds out" to him this or that physician.[15] That phenomenon alone has been enough to convince courts that hospitals could be enjoined in lawsuits against physicians to whom the hospital has awarded practice privileges. Under an agency theory of liability, courts reason that the hospital functions as the "apparent authority" for the people who work there, regardless of whether those people are salaried employees or independent contractors. Courts reason that as far as patients are concerned, it is ultimately "the hospital" that provides the services they receive and that the hospital could therefore be held liable for the torts of certain of the professionals who work there, even if the latter retain independent employment status.[16]

As legal scholars point out, though, the premise of agency liability seems to rest on the very questionable hypothesis that patients simply assume that any health professional who works in a hospital is an employee of that hospital.[17] When plaintiffs sue hospitals along with the hospital's independent contractor physician, courts virtually never ask plaintiffs to prove that they formulated and then relied on that false assumption.[18] Indeed, one wonders what difference it would make to most patients if, upon being admitted to a hospital, they are told that the surgeon who will be performing their procedure is not an employee of the hospital but an independent contractor. It is hard to imagine many patients responding, "Oh, well, that changes everything. I want a surgeon who is a salaried employee of the hospital." But if a physician's employment affiliation with the hospital is of little concern to most patients, it is hard to see why courts allow patients to enjoin hospitals primarily on the basis of a presumption courts believe patients make (i.e., that the physician is an employee of the hospital). And yet, even among hospitals that go to some lengths to inform their patients that the physicians taking care of them are not hospital employees, courts virtually always allow patient-plaintiffs to enjoin the hospital in the suit even though, as legal scholars Abraham and Weiler pointed out, the courts "would seem logically required to decline to impose liability when the hospital dispels that appearance."[19, p. 389]

A much more obvious reason, however, for a hospital to be held liable for the wrongs of its independent contractors is when the hospital knew or should have known that the professional in question presented a risk to patients that subsequently materialized.[20] Under a corporate liability theory, a hospital would certainly be held liable if it contracted with Dr. Williams to do surgery but failed to check Dr. Williams's credentials when he initially applied for surgical privileges and when doing so would have revealed he was never trained in surgery. Or if Dr. Williams had notoriously sloppy handwriting that occasionally resulted in mistaken medications, or if Dr. Williams was suspected of a drinking problem that no one in administration ever investigated or addressed. Just as obvious is the hospital's liability for failing to maintain or keep sterile the equipment Dr. Williams uses in surgery, or its complicity in failing to inform a patient that the real reason she needed an additional surgery two days after the first one is because Dr. Williams left a clamp in her abdomen. These are all obvious liability components of a healthcare organization that holds itself out to consumers as a provider of trustworthy and competently delivered services.

As such, hospitals can easily be (and commonly are) included in malpractice litigation against their staff regardless of whether staff are salaried or whether they independently contract their services with that hospital. Suppose, however, that hospitals or healthcare organizations simply configured their liability exposure into an all-embracing structure that absorbed an individual worker's liability for civil wrongdoing or tort. In other words, suppose a hospital or healthcare organization stood in for whatever civil wrongs its workers committed such that the individual would not be sued, only the organization. Might that phenomenon affect the disclosure of medical error in a morally favorable way and might it have other positive utilities as well?

Enterprise Liability and Medical Error Disclosure

Under an enterprise system of liability, the firm, organization, or corporation is the single defendant in a lawsuit.[21] Unlike the no-fault system we will discuss later, enterprise liability is a *fault-based* system so that plaintiffs who allege they have been wronged would not only have to prove they suffered harm but that the harm resulted from a defendant's failure to comply with the professional standard of care.[22] The point of the enterprise liability construct, however, is that the organization would stand as the sole bearer of liability so that its staff, especially its independently contracting physicians, would be spared the distasteful experience and financial encumbrances of being sued. How would this system work and what are its moral ramifications?

Enterprise liability would be financed by the professional who makes some sort of payment as a kind of malpractice premium to either the hospital or the managed care plan that contracts with him or her. This payment, whether in the form of a reduced fee for service or some kind of surcharge, would be the primary source for payouts to plaintiffs who prevail in their suits.[23] Now, there are numerous and immediate questions that this financial structure presents, such as whether hospitals might overcharge independent physicians, whether the deep-pocket aspect of enterprise liability might encourage more or higher awards, or whether enterprise liability might occur through legislative authorization or by contract.[24] I will only alert the reader to the more technical discussions. For now, I wish to focus on certain of the moral dimensions of enterprise liability.

First of all, if it is true that many if not most medical errors occur from system failure, then enterprise liability offers a more representative defendant in the form of the institution than the individual physician who, as we have seen, might have been set up for the error to occur. For any number of errors, especially wrong-side surgeries, wrong patient surgeries, and medication errors, it is virtually inevitable that multiple persons made multiple mistakes that allowed harm to occur.[25] Although the attending physician might continue to view him- or herself as the "captain of the ship," that metaphor has become an anachronism given the highly complex network of interdependencies that characterize a modern healthcare organization.[26] Consequently, an enterprise notion of liability posits a defendant who will often be more representative of the phenomenon that allowed a harm-causing error to occur. By presenting and adopting a definition of blame as collectivized and institutionalized, enterprise liability is more true to the nature of harm-causing error materialization than is the tort system we currently have.

Second, because individual healthcare professionals would not be sued under an enterprise construct, only the institution, the institution might be more encouraged to identify and remediate latent system problems.[27] To the extent that the institution collects premiums from individuals whose collective and inter-related efforts make for harm-causing errors, the institution would have an obvious incentive to institute systemic changes that reduce the frequency of errors and the harms resulting from them.

Legal scholars point out that although one of the aims of the tort system is deterrence, there is virtually no evidence that parties who are sued go on to substantially change their practice styles.[28] One reason for this is that most physicians who are sued are sued very infrequently. And because their malpractice carrier pays for any eventual settlement or jury award, neither the physician nor his or her hospital experiences an immediate or direct financial loss, unless the physician or hospital has assumed a deductible. Furthermore, a physician's malpractice premiums are not "experience rated" as is automobile insurance or individual health insurance, so the insured health professional usually does not pay a premium according to his or her individual risk history.[29] Rather, contemporary malpractice premium hikes reflect an overall industry phenomenon of higher costs that are recouped by passing them along as higher premiums to physician *groups*. Thus, neurosurgeons as a group will pay higher premiums than family practice physicians.

When the hospital itself is solely liable—especially if the hospital, as many currently do, insures itself and its doctors for an initial payout (and then purchases "stop-loss" insurance for settlements or awards higher than, say, $15 million)—the hospital would have more incentive to take an active interest in those latent system failures that facilitate error occurrences. Indeed, whereas the current tort model—wherein each of the multiple defendants has an attorney who is, after all, zealously advocating for that singular client and not the others—represents a fragmented approach to liability, enterprise liability accentuates a teamwork model, not only in instances of suit but also in advancing a more integrated approach to quality care and patient satisfaction.[30]

As such, a third advantage of enterprise liability consists in an organization's realization that remedying whatever unprofessional or unskilled behaviors exist among its staff is in its best interests. Gerald Hickson and his colleagues at Vanderbilt studied how the number of patient complaints against an individual physician is a powerful predictor of lawsuits against that individual and his or her employer hospital.[31] Under an enterprise liability construct, the hospital would have a greater incentive to identify those individuals and remedy their performance problems. If efforts at remediation fail, the hospital would have a powerful incentive to dismiss those staff or curtail their privileges.

The teamwork model that enterprise liability encourages may offer a fourth benefit: a more integrated, shared, and uniform practice of error disclosure. As we have seen from our case study, the disclosure of error at many hospitals is immensely dependent on the interpretational perspective and communication style of a small group of individuals. What counts as an error, whether the error was deemed to have caused harm, assessing the gravity of the harm, and then deciding on how expansive a conversation about an unanticipated outcome are usually decisions made and executed by a very small, often ad hoc committee. On the other hand, one often hears anecdotal reports of a patient being told "what happened" by multiple hospital personnel and then becoming bewildered and angered when there are informational gaps and inconsistencies. As we also saw in a previous chapter, there is good reason to think this probably leads to numerous lawsuits wherein a patient's attending physician omits information in an initial discussion that, later on, is intimated or outright supplied by someone else. In conversations wherein the stakes are high, enterprise liability might well encourage a more reflective, practiced, and uniform approach to what is said and how it is said. Such an approach to error disclosure, because it will be institutionally mediated, might more consistently reflect a patient-centered sensibility. Of course, because an enterprise approach would not witness an individual physician's being sued, it is fair to speculate that whatever relief accrues from transferring liability entirely to the institution would encourage more truthful error disclosure.

Conclusion: Enterprise Liability. In 1993, President Clinton proposed an enterprise liability construct in his wide-ranging health reform plan that was defeated by the Physician Insurer Association of America, which doubtlessly worried that such a plan would obviate the need for physicians to carry insurance and therefore toll the demise of individual carriers.[32] Sadly, over the last 10 years, many of those carriers have indeed gone out of business, but not because of a declining need for their product. The problem has been that the product itself has become too expensive and too risky to finance.[33] It is suggested that an enterprise system as well as the no-fault system we will soon examine offer certain advantages over the current tort system. Perhaps the most prominent resistance to an enterprise system is a fear of the unknown. True, there is concern over whether settlements and awards might increase under an enterprise system because the shining and structurally imposing modern-day hospital might seem to represent a bottomless well of money for potential plaintiffs. There is also concern about how a physician who has multiple affiliations (or none) would align him- or herself with an institution and whether that institution ought be a hospital or a health plan organization. And there are concerns about what the enterprise construct would cost, although with one defendant rather than multiple defendants, overall defense and administrative costs should diminish. Last, physicians worry that the institution to which they would pay premiums might gouge them with excessively high rates, although economists counter that marketplace competition among hospitals ought to result in reasonable premiums or surcharges.[34]

Advocates for the enterprise construct seemed fundamentally attracted to the congruence of the construct with the reality of medical errors and how the construct might positively advance patient-centered goals by encouraging a more consistent and integrated approach to increasing the quality of care. Perhaps it is time to replace the "captain of the ship" metaphor with the "aircraft carrier" metaphor, wherein anyone on deck has the authority to call off the mission. That kind of shared responsibility is more representative of clinical operations in today's hospitals and encourages a liability construct that reflects it. What follows is a discussion of a more dramatic construct that also seeks to advance the same quality and patient-centered goals as enterprise liability: namely, the no-fault construct.

No-Fault

Whereas enterprise liability requires that plaintiffs prove fault or negligence, no-fault insurance, as its name implies, imposes no such requirement.[35] All that is necessary to secure compensation under a no-fault system is for a patient-claimant to show that he or she suffered an avoidable and significant adversity while in the hospital and that the adversity was caused by some hospital operation or one or more of the hospital's personnel.[36] Assuming that the claimant's adversity rises to whatever severity threshold exists to trigger compensation, the injured individual would then receive some sort of payment consistent with his or her medical expenses, lost time from work, or level of disability occurring from the injury. An award for pain and suffering might also be available, but all payments made to a claimant would be calculated according to a pre-set, actuarial formula in contrast to the tort system's referring that determination to a jury. Just like workers' compensation, which is another type of no-fault, the system would be designed and administered by state government.[37]

A no-fault system thus takes the liability relief provided to individual professionals under an enterprise system a considerable step further. Under no-fault, *negligence becomes a nonissue* because payments are not determined on that basis.[38] Rather, a group of experts would most likely be impaneled to hear allegations and determine whether or not a claim is meritorious. If it is, compensation would be awarded in a fairly rapid fashion according to whatever payment schedule the state adopts. Moreover, and very unlike lump-sum jury awards in tort litigation, compensation through no-fault would be distributed in periodic payments as needed by the claimant.[39]

Under no-fault, the truly or essentially "malpracticing" physician would be one who resorted to wanton, intentional, and egregious wrongdoing, representing a marked contrast to the current experience of malpractice as a failure to conform to the professional standard of care.[40] While it might (or might not) be the case that each health professional who enrolls in a no-fault arrangement would have his or her premiums adjusted according to the number of claims made against him or her, just like motorists involved in auto accidents, the onerous nature of the fault-finding process of the malpractice suit would disappear. Health professionals would largely be spared the humiliation and irritation of the tort process as well as anxiety over whether or not their insurance will be able to cover whatever compensation the claimant eventually receives.[41]

Indeed, a huge advantage over the current tort system claimed by advocates of no-fault is that the former not only witnesses too many frivolous lawsuits, but it also does not compensate enough victims who have suffered a negligently caused adverse outcome. A widely quoted finding from the 1991 Harvard Malpractice Study is that for every eight individuals who suffer injuries caused by negligence, only one files a claim, primarily because the damages that could reasonably be projected from the other seven are insufficient to interest a plaintiff attorney's taking the case.[42] One must realize that whereas defense attorneys in tort litigation are usually paid on an hourly basis by the malpractice insurer, attorneys who represent plaintiffs are paid only if there is some settlement or jury award. Commonly, their share of that award is from 33 to 40 percent. But if the individual alleging malpractice can show only a modest level of injury that would translate into a similarly modest award, he or she might be unable to find an attorney willing to take the case. Alternatively, an attorney might not wish to proceed with a case because he or she deems the burden of proof—especially having to show that the injury the patient sustained was due to negligence—too high.

No-fault, however, would allow more modest awards to come forward as well as reduce the claimant's burden of proof. Hence, there would probably be a substantial increase in claims.[43] Proponents of no-fault nevertheless believe that a substantial rise in claims and payouts would not financially overwhelm no-fault's capacity to compensate injured persons because they believe that the overall costs of the no-fault system would be substantially less than the current tort system.[44] No-fault advocates point out that attorney fees on both sides would be much lower than they presently are and that a governmentally administered system would eventually be streamlined and its practices made uniform. As such, no-fault advocates claim that more of the system's expenses would go directly into the pockets of persons who have a rightful claim to that money, that administrative inefficiencies would be drastically reduced, that payments to claimants would occur much more rapidly than the current tort system allows, and that as the system evolves and large databases develop, there would be substantial empirical data to assist the system in making just and fair compensation decisions.[45]

Two No-Fault Systems

In the 1980s, Virginia and Florida implemented no-fault systems for catastrophic neonatal cases.[46] Although neither state has a sufficient number of yearly cases to allow confident assessments of their operational quality—with Virginia averaging about 4 filings a year and Florida about 26 and only a fraction of either resulting in payment—it is worthwhile to note a few items about their administration, membership, practices, compensation history, and user satisfaction.

The programs were launched to enable physicians to have insurance. They are funded mainly through a $5,000 yearly assessment on physicians who choose to participate (and virtually all do) as well as a $250 per year assessment on physicians who do not. In Florida, all prospective patients, who are all pregnant women, must be given notice well in advance of their delivery date as to whether or not their physician participates in the no-fault system so that they can choose to be served by a nonparticipating physician. The reason this is a crucial consideration is that these programs are intended to be "exclusive remedies," meaning that tort claims are barred unless injury was caused "in bad faith, with malicious purpose or in willful and wanton disregard of human rights."[47, p. 84] If rejected for no-fault, however, a claimant can resort to a traditional tort remedy.

The claim itself must meet a threshold of eligibility (or harmfulness). In Virginia, that threshold allows only, "extremely serious, birth related neurological injuries—cases where a live infant is permanently disabled and in need of assistance in all activities of daily living."[48, p. 90] In Florida, the infant must be "permanently and substantially mentally and physically impaired."[49, p. 90] Children whose disabilities are caused genetically or manifest a congenital abnormality are explicitly excluded as well as children in Virginia whose disability results from maternal substance abuse. In Virginia, benefits are limited to pecuniary loss as well as necessary and reasonable expenses connected with medical, residential, and custodial care. Attorneys are paid on an hourly basis.[50]

Hearings are public as are the formal records, including medical records. Proceedings occur before the no-fault commission. Medical reviews of claims are performed by physicians selected by authorities not connected with the programs. Only patients of providers who participate in the no-fault program can file claims, and only participating physicians are protected by no-fault compensation. Almost all obstetricians in both states participate in the no-fault programs.[51]

Treating physicians whose patients receive compensation do not witness rate increases as the "programs make no attempt to assess individual physician performance because they operate under no-fault standards."[52, p. 103] Furthermore, the National Practitioner Data Bank—which is the national informational repository of a physician's malpractice and disciplinary history and which is checked when that physician applies anywhere for privileges—is not notified of no-fault determinations as it would be if a malpractice carrier settled a case or made compensation to a plaintiff per a jury award.[53]

Although claims in the no-fault system are not filed any faster than they are in tort cases, no-fault claims are settled in about 25 percent of the time (six months versus two years). The no-fault system has no apparent effect on a physician's practice patterns.[54]

No-Fault and Errors

I have been unable to locate any data on how these no-fault programs affect how a health professional communicates error to patients. But even if there were such data, any generalizations from it would be problematic because the cases are so few in number. That is indeed unfortunate because it would be interesting to observe how error disclosure would be affected if error was not a component of the claimant's burden of proof. Is it the case, for example, that no-fault physicians would not feel they needed to admit error and therefore would not disclose because it would be inconsequential to the claimant's case? Or would the fact that no-fault relieves physicians from the threat of malpractice litigation make them more inclined toward greater expansiveness in their discussion of what happened?

An even more fundamental question than error disclosure concerns the extent to which no-fault would or would not curtail the commission of errors themselves. Experience with automobile no-fault indicates a slight increase in the number of accidents in no-fault states, which some scholars attribute to no-fault engendering a slightly less careful approach among motorists because such accidents go down as "blameless."[55] Would an analogous situation develop in medicine, wherein professionals might commit more errors if they no longer feared malpractice litigation?

Indeed, because claimants would bring cases in the absence of fault, would professionals become more blasé about adverse outcomes in general? It is possible that many more cases would be filed under a no-fault approach than currently exist in tort litigation because no-fault filings would not be encumbered by an attorney's concern about the extent of damages or proving that negligence caused the injury. In fact, one of the prominent fears surrounding no-fault is that there would be so many claimants that the system would ultimately become too expensive.[56] Moreover, while plaintiffs in the current system will want to impress the judge and jury with the extent and gravity of the harms they allege having suffered from negligence, no-fault claimants might instead be tempted to inordinately prolong whatever harm they have sustained, because no-fault benefits are paid out over a period of time and according to the claimant's need.[57] Would claimants, as sometimes happens in workers' compensation cases, malinger? Would moral responsibility on either side of the provider-patient relationship wane? Would physicians no longer practice disciplined care because the penalties for failure to do so have declined? And would patients, if harmed while receiving medical care, prolong their disability and time away from work as much as possible and become free-riders on no-fault resources?

It seems to me that the benefits of no-fault are more geared toward remediating various dysfunctions in the current tort system than creating a mechanism that has a salutary effect on superior management of medical errors. No-fault proposes to distribute compensation more efficiently among persons unexpectedly harmed by health professionals and to reach a larger proportion of injured patients than the current tort system does. Also, because tort litigation can take years to complete and the malpractice marketplace is dramatically affected by an insurer's investments, actuarialization of premiums often lags behind the insurer's actual losses, which eventually causes dramatic premium hikes. No-fault payouts, on the other hand, are much more temporally proximate to the filings themselves and hence promise more accurate and less volatile pricing.[58]

Conclusion: No-fault. If enterprise liability presents an anxiety-provoking departure from the traditional way of doing business, no-fault seems only for the very brave at heart. Not only does it provoke considerable speculation about maintaining quality care, but the construct itself would doubtlessly encounter constitutional challenges. One that looms large would be whether or not hospitals and physicians would enjoy inappropriate bargaining power under no fault when drawing patients into the scheme.[59] The woman who wants Dr. Smith to deliver her baby might pay little attention to the nature of waiving her rights in tort, which include a jury trial, if Dr. Smith works exclusively in a no-fault environment. Has she, by virtue of her dependency on Dr. Smith, been unreasonably coerced into an arrangement that is ultimately to Dr. Smith's benefit? These and other empirically based questions on the extent to which no-fault would make healthcare more or less safe suggest that a thoroughgoing no-fault system in medicine seems a long way off, should it ever materialize.

Introduction

Some years before the Institute of Medicine's report *To Err Is Human* appeared, patient safety researchers emphasized the liabilities of blame and punishment of health professionals who commit errors.[60] Their position, as discussed in Chapter 1, was that many if not most harm-causing errors occur because of faults in the care delivery system. System failures occur when personnel find themselves in situations that might dispose them to harm-causing errors—such as when, for example, personnel are assigned procedures to perform before they are adequately trained, or when the system fails to intercept an error that eventually causes harm, such as occurred in the Willie King wrong leg amputation case.

This position accepts human fallibility as frankly inevitable and repudiates the perfectionist model as hopelessly unrealistic and inconsistent with patient safety objectives.[61] While systems should obviously institute mechanisms that reduce the number of errors, "imperfectionist" models accept the notion that the variables that can contribute to an adverse clinical outcome (ranging from the degree of a patient's compliance with his treatment regimen to the way a physician's mood on any given day might affect his or her attentiveness to clinical details) are too numerous to control; that treatment decisions often rely on multiple sources of information, among which certain ones are less accurate or reliable than others; that professional judgments will frequently be made and acted upon in the absence of adequate information; that much of the care process witnesses an extremely complex operator-to-technology interface where breakdowns on either side of that interface commonly occur; that care personnel managing a single case might have varying levels of competence and familiarity with the treatment plan; that the risk awareness and risk aversiveness of different care providers might predispose them to recommend vastly different action plans; and that much of healthcare occurs in stressful, fluid, unstable, dynamic, and unpredictable situations whose contours can change more rapidly than the system's response capacity.[62]

Consequently, organizations that are convinced of the validity of the systemic approach to error will not only resist blaming the error operators, but when errors occur, will have mechanisms that help involved staff therapeutically manage whatever feelings of guilt, shame, inadequacy, or horror they might experience. As we have already seen, professionals involved in errors frequently experience immense anguish that can be devastating. What is more, staff not involved in the error might shy away from the involved personnel almost as though the latter have contracted a contagious case of "erroritis."[63] The possibility that staff involved in error might be professionally abandoned by their peers should prompt organizations to implement support and counseling interventions, such as are commonly available from employee assistance programs.

Such organizations will resist blaming and punishing error operators for another reason. Because these organizations are convinced that patient safety is best promoted by systemic changes and that harm-causing errors are largely explained by system failures, these facilities recognize that a policy of blame and punishment in the event of error compromises system improvement.[64] The individual who knows he or she has committed an error but anticipates that an error report will result in some sort of organizational penalty will be less inclined to report the error. Deprived of that report, the organization is unable to uncover, investigate, and remediate those systemic elements that might explain the error's occurrence. If a system failure was indeed at the root of the error and especially at the root of the harm it caused, then a "blame and punish" response to error diminishes the chance that the error will be reported and simultaneously improves the chances that the system failure will remain unchanged.

Furthermore, it is eminently fair to say that blame and punishment not only discourage error reports but also error disclosure. If the costs of calling attention to an error are perceived as too high, human nature will be powerfully tempted to conceal it. While it is not illogical for an organization that employs a "blame and punish" response to error to also insist on error disclosure, it is rather unimaginable that the employee who resists error reporting because of an organization's promise of penalties will nevertheless disclose the error to the harmed party. On the other hand, while it is not illogical for an organization that maintains a "blameless and nonpunitive" policy to also maintain a policy of error concealment or obfuscation toward the harmed party, it is much more likely that error disclosure will occur in those environments where error reporting is empathically supported and facilitated. Obviously, the more that professional and personal stigmatizations are removed from error occurrence, the more inclined persons involved in error will be to report and disclose the error in a patient-centered fashion.

It would be splendid to end this section with this understanding of blame and punishment as antiquated remnants of a less informed, needlessly brutal era of risk and personnel management. Consider the following case, however, which I pieced together from a number of risk management horror stories:

> *Surgeon Jones makes no attempt to conceal his alcohol consumption. Several of his fellow surgeons tried to have friendly chats with him about his drinking, but he denies he has a problem.*
>
> *One day, Dr. Jones seems inebriated during a surgery, and a surgical clamp is left in the patient's abdomen, which perforates the patient's bowel. In securing consent to the additional surgery to remove the clamp and repair the bowel, the patient and his family are only told that the second surgery is required because of "complications" from the first one. During the surgery, Jones says to the operating room staff, "These things happen, but at this hospital we support one another."*
>
> *Nurse Goodheart, who has been newly hired and is aware of the harm-causing error, is very bothered by all of this and speaks with her supervisor. The supervisor appears extremely uncomfortable as Goodheart relates her story but advises her to consult with risk management, which she does. Risk*

management, in turn, tells Goodheart not to put anything in writing, and that they will take care of everything.

A few weeks later, Goodheart is dismissed because of "unanticipated budget constraints." She learns some months later that nothing ever came of her reporting Dr. Jones, that his drinking persists, and that the harmed patient required multiple hospitalizations in the meantime. Nurse Goodheart calls a very capable malpractice attorney and tells him all she knows. In subsequent months, all the sordid details of the case emerge. When hospital administrators are asked why they took no action against Dr. Jones, they reply that their new organizational initiative is to sustain a "blameless and nonpunitive" environment.

David Marx, who explored the development of a "just" healthcare culture and whose work I will discuss below, remarked, "I am aware of no organization in the world, even those professing a 'blame-free' disciplinary system that will not discipline an individual who has been reckless toward the safety of others." [65, p.] Similarly James Reason remarked:

> A "no-blame" culture is neither feasible nor desirable. A small proportion of human unsafe acts are egregious (for example, substance abuse, reckless non-compliance, sabotage and so on) and warrant sanctions, severe ones in some cases. A blanket amnesty on all unsafe acts would lack credibility in the eyes of the workforce. More importantly, it would be seen to oppose natural justice. [66, p. 195]

Certainly, a non-blaming, non-corrective response to Dr. Jones is grossly irresponsible and morally cowardly. But what does it actually mean to "blame" someone? Is blaming someone for a harm different from holding him or her responsible for that harm? And if there are certain acts that are categorically blameworthy but others that are not, how does one tell the difference? Indeed, how does all this bear on the disclosure of error and the imposition of punishment?

Understanding and Assessing Responsibility

A philosophically familiar characterization of harm holds it to be "a setback of interest." [67] On that account, a judge who hands down a life sentence to a serial rapist is clearly "responsible" for harming him—after all, the rapist will spend the rest of his life in very inhospitable surroundings per the court's sentencing. Assuming, however, that the judge did not violate any of the norms and dictates of justice, he would only be responsible for, but not to "blame" for, the harm he caused the rapist because our moral intuitions tell us the judge acted morally and reasonably.

A standard account of responsibility would at least include the following. For individual X to be held responsible for phenomenon Y's occurrence (whether Y is beneficial, harmful, or neutral as it relates to someone's welfare), X must at least:

1) Cause Y to happen or set in motion events that cause Y to happen

2) Knowingly understand that his actions may result in Y

3) Mean or intend for Y to happen

4) Understand the moral dimensions and implications of Y

5) Behave freely and voluntarily.[68]

A little reflection on these criteria shows why ascribing responsibility needs to be very contextual but that it can nevertheless be highly problematic.

First of all, if responsibility entails playing a causal role in Y, then responsibility can admit degrees per the extent to which one or more persons actively contribute to Y's occurrence. The surgeon who fails to close a suture adequately is entirely responsible for that error, but causal responsibility for Willie King's wrong-side surgery was shared by any number of persons. Each one was "partially" responsible because each of their errors played causal roles in the harm Mr. King sustained. So, here the problem is identifying persons who actually "contributed" to the harm-causing error and then assessing levels or degrees of responsibility for each.

Second, while the nature and possibility of freely willed behavior have been debated since the birth of Western philosophy, the assumption that certain of our actions can occur against our will is widely accepted as a mitigating factor in assessing responsibility. Consider, for example, the case of a sleep-deprived resident surgeon who is told in no uncertain terms by the chief of surgery to scrub for an operation. The resident feels that he cannot refuse the chief's request. So, if the resident falls asleep while standing over the surgical site and "face plants" into it, determining his responsibility might elicit any number of interpretations that diminish his responsibility. Some might argue that the resident felt coerced into participating in the procedure; or that his sleep deprivation may have clouded his judgment as to whether or not he should have acquiesced to the chief's request; or that the chief should be held responsible for this adverse incident because he failed to assess the resident's alertness.

Third, gauging responsibility with any degree of precision becomes even more complicated when we consider the role of intentionality in responsible behavior. Clearly, the resident did not mean to, want to, or choose to collapse into the patient's body during the surgery; yet, the resident did indeed intend his participation in the surgery. The physician whose sloppy handwriting is misread such that it leads to a medication error clearly *caused* his poor handwriting, but *did not cause* its misinterpretation. He intended it to appear as it did because he did not change or improve it, but he did not intend for it to be misread. And he certainly did not intend for the patient to get the wrong medication. The plot thickens further when certain errors appear in the early stages of the error trajectory (e.g., the poorly written order), while others appear at the sharp end (e.g., the nurse who administers the wrong medication). "Sharp-end" errors often appear much more dramatic than blunt-end ones, yet the blunt-end error might be more dramatic, shocking, or egregious.

These very sketchy observations nevertheless show why assigning responsibility for Y—regardless of whether the welfare impact of Y was good, bad, or indifferent—can be immensely problematic. The categories of causality, comprehension, intentionality, and volition might admit degrees, but no explicit metric is available to determine those degrees with any precision. While it would be immensely welcome to have such measures for holding professionals responsible for their actions, human intentions and interactions can be so complex and our scientific capacity to measure and evaluate those intersections so wanting that the best efforts to assess responsibility, especially when things go wrong, can leave considerable room for debate or disagreement. Furthermore, in instances where multiple persons might be held responsible for an adversity, one cannot ignore the possibility that some of them will inject their own biased and self-interested interpretations into the event analysis. We will return to this discussion later. For now, though, we will turn attention to the phenomenon of blame.

Blame

In the midst of an argument, Jack unexpectedly and without any real provocation throws two punches at Jim. Jim deflects both blows and forcefully pushes Jack away. Jack loses his balance, falls, strikes his head on the way down, and lands unconscious. Is Jim "responsible" for Jack's concussion? Well, Jim certainly caused Jack to fall backward, but conversely, Jack's starting the scuffle meant that he had a causal role in his concussion as well. Still, Jim did not have to fight back. And while Jim might not have intended for Jack to sustain a concussion, if Jim acted voluntarily and recognized the possibility that Jack might sustain an injury, we might hold Jim at least somewhat responsible for Jack's concussion. Yet, assuming Jim only intended to defend himself and not harm Jack, we would resist "blaming" Jim for Jack's injury. Why?

Because blaming X for Y takes X considerably beyond responsibility for Y. To blame means that X *wronged* whomever it was that experienced Y and wronging, as we have already seen, is more than harming. If harming is understood as an "interest setback," then persons are harmed all the time and every day. I suffer harm if I break a shoelace as I hurriedly get dressed for work; am delayed in getting to work because I must scrape ice off my car's windshield on a bitterly cold morning; arrive at work only to learn that the coffee machine is broken; and then realize I left my reading glasses at home.[69]

Wronging, however, means violating another's rights or harming him or her in a way that is socially intolerable.[70] Importantly, human beings can be responsible for harming one another *without* wronging them: the employer who is forced to lay off workers in order to trim expenses; the professor who fails a student who cannot learn material; even the health professional whose diagnostic tests might cause a patient considerable pain and discomfort. But in none of these instances has the harm-bearer suffered an authentic wrong or *injustice,* such as would occur from the employer who discriminates among his employees, the professor who grades in an arbitrary and capricious manner, or the physician who covertly engages in sadism.[71]

Blame means to direct an accusation of wrongdoing at someone, where wronging tokens the assumption of at least a moral and virtually always a legal debt.[72] If the accusation of wronging is valid, then the blameworthy individual has caused another to suffer a loss or setback, which his or her society requires be amended or remedied. Now sometimes, the victim of the wronging might relieve the debt by forgiving the victimizer, as we saw in Chapter 5. As a benevolence-based response to wronging, forgiveness dismisses (although it does not necessarily forget) the circumstances of the blame, and relieves the victimizer of his or her debt repayment. Punishment, on the other hand, is the outcome of a justice-based response that is predicated on a valid act of blaming.[73]

Very importantly, because all harm-causing errors are wrongs and not just harms, *all acts of harm-causing errors are potentially blamable from the harmed party's perspective.* This explains why the disclosure of harm-causing error is morally obligatory. Because the patient has been wronged, he or she has the right to have some say in determining what kind of "debt release" might occur, that is, whether it takes the form of some kind of punishment ranging from an apology to prosecution, or whether the debt be released without punishment. Disclosure of error acknowledges the harmed individual's right to decide whether or not to blame and punish.

Establishing a blameless and nonpunitive environment, on the other hand, is a purely internal, institutional consideration that derives from the moral relationship between the institution and its employees. As observed in a previous chapter, the institution obviously cannot hold the erring professional blameless *in relation to the harmed party* because the institution cannot speak for the party who has been wronged. Thus, for those who conceal errors, the rather common rationalization that "The patient will be too upset to learn this," or "Nothing will bring the patient back to the way he or she was," is ethically obtuse because it dismisses the patient's right to fashion a response to the wrong he or she has suffered. The patient must be informed of the error because he or she wields the right to determine whether or to what degree the wrongdoers will be blamed and punished.

While an error disclosure policy speaks to the institution's understanding of its relationship between itself and its patients, a "blameless and nonpunitive" response policy will define the institution's posture only between itself and its employees. On what moral bases, then, might the institution blame and impose punishment on its erring staff?

Blaming: Some Preliminary Considerations

If blaming connotes wronging and a patient's suffering a harm-causing error is an instance of wronging, might there be *levels or degrees of wronging* that determine the blamability and punishability of error operators? In a thoughtful paper on developing a just healthcare culture, David Marx explores various types of error that might inform the elements of a "blamability gradient."[74] I will discuss Marx's model and supplement it with additional material.

While Marx discusses four types of errors, I will collapse his distinctions into three error types that might inform an institution's calculation of blame and punishment. The first error type is simply one of unintentional error in conjunction with an unintentional process violation that may or may not cause harm. (In fact, an intentional or unintentional process violation is itself a technical error, which can make for confusion in the error analysis.) The second type involves erring conduct in conjunction with an intentional violation of care standards, again regardless of whether it causes harm or not. The third type consists of reckless conduct, with or without harm as a result.

As with the above examples, the phenomenon of intentionality looms large in this analysis because blame models that are based only on outcome are, as Marx and others correctly observe, highly problematic. For example, I am familiar with a medical error wherein an order for 10 units of oxycodone was misread as 100 units, which the patient received. The patient, however, was well over six feet tall and weighed about 300 pounds. When the oxycodone wore off with no adverse effects, he remarked to the nurse that "that medicine was the best I ever had in my life and I'd sure appreciate it if the doctor wrote me a prescription for it so I could get some at home."

While this story never fails to elicit a laugh when I tell it, suppose the patient was very frail and elderly. In that scenario, the dose could have been lethal. But suppose that in the two scenarios, the error trajectories that ended with 100 units of the narcotic being given were utterly identical with the only difference being the patients' physiology. Because *health professionals should have only moral responsibility for what they can reasonably control and none for what they cannot reasonably control,* moral culpability should involve only the error trajectory itself and its potential for harm. Although the health professional in the first oxycodone instance would probably thank the gods for her good fortune while the one in the second would be utterly devastated, *a morally objective* institutional analysis of either error would *omit* the actual outcome and focus on the moments of the error pathway itself because the outcome cannot be controlled.[75]

Admittedly, that omission is psychologically very hard to do. Yet, the erring professional's *luck* should not be a moral factor in his or her bearing the blame for an unintentional error. For example, prescription errors do occur but are usually intercepted before patients are harmed because a significant amount of time elapses after the order is written, so a hospital's defense mechanisms can check and recheck the order. The otherwise competent surgeon, however, who fails to suture a surgical wound properly does not have the good fortune to have his or her error wind its way through multiple layers of patient safety defenses. His or her area of practice witnesses a tight temporal proximity between the error and whatever harm it might cause. A blameless-nonpunitive policy will therefore recognize that an otherwise competent surgeon should not be blamed for a suture error because the policy stipulates that the surgeon does not have the good fortune to benefit from the kind of harm protection that another physician does who, for example, sloppily writes out a medication order.

Of course, an error committed by any physician can have graver consequences than an error committed by a hospital ethicist. But this does not mean that we blame the former more than the latter; rather, it means that we hold the former to a higher level of competence, especially per his or her training and eventual licensure or board certification. The point remains that once an individual demonstrates adequacy and competence in his or her profession, his or her random unintentional errors that do not demonstrate an intentional violation of standard organizational safety procedures should not be blamable because absolutely no one is immune from error commission.

A blameless/nonpunitive policy also resists blame in instances of unintentional harm-causing error regardless of whether the error was committed by a single person or was the work of multiple persons. This is important because our natural impulse is to hold a single-point, harm-causing error operator more blamable than when multiple operators commit discrete errors that ultimately link up to cause a disaster. But again, this is a circumstantial element of the accident occurrence that should not morally affect our evaluation of an individual error operator's blamability. Where multiple errors and error operators link up to cause a disaster, each error contributor nevertheless makes a discrete and focal error. *Each constitutes a single-point failure in the harm trajectory chain.* The fact that the cumulative effect of these errors ultimately allows harm to occur does not morally distinguish this scenario from one wherein a seemingly discrete error by a sole error operator was the sole cause of harm. The point is that once the error leaves an operator's control, only the contingencies of the situation determine whether it might be reasonably intercepted or not, and cause harm or not.

This raises a last point: While the overwhelming number of medical errors are discrete and committed by single individuals, it is especially unjust to blame a single individual just because he or she is the most *conspicuous* of the error operators. Thus, our shock at Dr. Anesthesiologist's error and subsequent behavior in Chapter 4 is understandable. But had a root cause analysis been performed that showed how the malfunction of the operating table's gears, the problem with the X-ray cassette, and the suspension of the alarms on the monitoring equipment all contributed to the catastrophe, Dr. Anesthesiologist would appear as only one of any number of error operators.

While all health professionals err, the ability to control the error's vector is an organizational or situational phenomenon and not one over which the individual error operator necessarily exerts adequate control. The physician who writes an erroneous prescription does not control the defense layers through which the order proceeds but benefits by their potential for error detection. The surgeon who errs in suturing tissue does not have the luxury of such protection but must hope to be able to remedy his error without the end result seriously harming the patient. So long as they are unintentional, do not additionally and intentionally violate standard procedures, and are committed by otherwise competent and dedicated staff, neither instance should augur blame on the error operators.

Errors and Process Violations

I have advanced the idea that blamability tokens an indebtedness that one incurs toward whomever he or she has wronged, and that punishment is the form that indebtedness generally assumes unless the wrong is forgiven. Because patients who have been harmed by medical error have also been wronged, they must be informed about the error so as to determine how the debt they are owed might be repaid or relieved. Thus, the truthful and honest delivery of that information is an essential moral component in dispatching the institution's responsibility toward those patients who have been harmed by errors. But what does this model of blamability/punishment *imply about an institution's relationship* with its employees? In other words, if an employer is going to "blame" an employee for wrongdoing, what does blamability mean in that organizational circumstance? In what way, according to our model of moral indebtedness, does the employee "owe" his or her employer organization, and what is the moral purpose or utility of punishment in such a situation?

The answers, I believe, run along the following lines. Human beings inevitably make errors as a result of having a brain with a highly evolved neocortex. Consequently, it is unreasonable for an institution to insist that its employees act errorlessly. What is reasonable, however, is that the institution design and implement patient safety practices and policies in caring for patients. What is also reasonable, indeed obligatory, is that institutions disseminate these patient safety practices to the relevant staff and ensure the staff have reasonably absorbed and learned that instruction. Once that is accomplished, it is perfectly legitimate for the organization to hold its employees to those practices as part of the organization's promise to the public that patients will not be exposed to substandard care. Obviously, patient safety practices reside in the same domain as standard-of-care practices. A patient safety admonition to nurses to never "borrow" Patient Jones's medicine to give to Patient Smith is as much a standard-of-care measure as a physician who refrains from operating on a patient whose blood pressure is inordinately and uncontrollably high. The health professional, then, who knows and attempts to abide by patient safety protocols and care standards and still errs does so unintentionally. Ordinarily, we cannot blame him or her. But the health professional who knowingly violates these standards in connection with error—indeed, such a violation itself counts as a technical error—may be blamable because he or she knowingly and intentionally breached his or her pledge to the institution, and to the patients the institution serves, to act in accordance with patient safety measures.[76]

I say "may" be blamable because, as the discussion above shows, there might be a host of mitigating circumstances whereby a professional's blamability can be contained. Suppose, for example, that the sleepless resident in the above scenario knowingly violated a policy that was designed for the safety of patients, such as the 80-hour rule. The resident might offer compelling justifications for his violation by identifying factors that facilitated or even encouraged the infraction, e.g., the resident's interpreting the chief surgeon's request for his participation as a quasi-command that could not be refused without repercussions, or the fact that the 80-hour rule is regarded at this hospital as hogwash. Common factors that affect blamability include whether or not the erring professional was adequately made aware of the fact that he or she committed a process violation (i.e., made a technical error because organizational safety standards were violated); whether or not the professional was induced to make the error because of a system flaw; or whether or not the professional knowingly violated policy because he or she believed that doing so was for the patient's welfare.[77] In other words, it is possible that extenuating or mitigating circumstances are present that might reduce an individual's blamability for an intentional process violation. Marx offers a provocative example:

> *A new transfusion service phlebotomist is on the early morning shift drawing samples on the hospital floor. She checks Ms. Jones's requisition and armband before she draws her samples.*
>
> *Ms. Jones is really annoyed about the bright lights the phlebotomist has turned on, and the phlebotomist is trying to placate Ms. Jones by turning them off quickly. She knows that there is a strict procedure to label tubes at the bedside, but as she has already positively identified the patient, and as this is the only set of tubes she has, she decides to label the tubes at the nurse's station.*
>
> *She lays the tubes down at the nurse's station and begins labeling. However, a nurse comes to the nurse's station with an unlabeled tube of blood and lays it down nearby. Not noticing this, the phlebotomist mistakenly thinks one of her tubes has rolled away. She picks up the nurse's tube and also labels it with Ms. Jones's information.*
>
> *Ms. Jones is a new patient and her blood type is unknown. The mislabeled tube is used to type and cross units for her. Ms. Jones has a moderately severe transfusion reaction when the first unit is being transfused.*[78, p. 9]

So, here the phlebotomist knowingly violated a patient safety measure and thus committed an intentional, technical error that unfortunately causes harm. Assume that the hospital can then impose various degrees of punishment. For example, on an ascending scale of repercussions: the phlebotomist might be charged with explaining and apologizing for the error to the patient (which would be morally required of someone from the organization in any case); an administrative reprimand added to the phlebotomist's personnel file; a suspension from work without pay; or dismissal. How severe should the penalty be?

The answer should be based on the phlebotomist's intention while committing the error, coupled with whatever the organizational punishment *is designed to accomplish*. While the phlebotomist cannot deny that she knowingly violated policy, notice that she might very well defend her action by saying that she did so out of concern for the patient's comfort. The patient's complaint about the bright lights the phlebotomist turned on to check the patient's armband and label the tubes is hardly unreasonable. The phlebotomist might therefore argue that she violated policy for a beneficently based reason—namely, to reduce the patient's discomfort even though the discomfort was caused by organizational policy.

Imagine a similar scenario wherein the tube labeling takes place at the nurse's station, except that no overt errors occur. This nevertheless counts as a technical error in the form of an intentional process violation. Further suppose that the phlebotomist asks to be present at the next supervisory, patient safety, or ethics committee meeting of the hospital and frankly tells the committee of her process violation and the fact that she and other phlebotomists constantly hear patients complain about blood draws early in the morning under bright lights. One can easily imagine a patient-centered committee deliberating and then recommending that phlebotomists be supplied with small flash-lights that they might wear around their wrists to preclude the problem of the bright lights. The interesting moral aspect of that recommendation involves the recognition that a system improvement can eliminate the temptation to violate a safety measure and that a system inadequacy, that is, not using more patient-friendly illumination, facilitates the process violation.

Risk managers are all too aware of how professionals sometimes cut corners and vio-late patient safety measures. Consider, for example, professionals performing proce-dures for which they are untrained or without supervision; the ethical notoriety of per-forming a "slow" code; the failure to "read back and verify" physician orders given telephonically; the failure to resterilize during an operation if the sterile field was bro-ken; the failure to monitor a patient adequately; or the failure to spell out medication names or dosages and instead use confusing abbreviations. Note, however, that some of these examples might admit rationales that could offset or reduce the professional's blamability because the professional might argue that complying with the patient safety protocol in a specific instance seriously compromised patient comfort or care. What is morally obvious is that when the professional who intentionally errs produces a roundly convincing justification for his or her process violation such that it was clearly per-formed in the patient's best interest, a knee-jerk blaming and punishing response seems problematic because *the only goal of organizational punishment ought to be deterrence.*[79]

Suppose in the imagined scenario where the phlebotomist addresses the patient safety committee on her intentional error, a member of the committee insists that the phlebotomist should receive a modest punishment for her admitted rule violation. What would that punishment accomplish? The institution that punishes the phlebotomist just to impress the employee with its corporate displeasure is simply sadistic. The effect of punishment in this instance might well be to cause the employee to blindly follow rules and to elevate an unquestioning obedience to those rules above all else, especially patient comfort or satisfaction. Indeed, Marx notes the phenomenon of malicious com-pliance "where a disgruntled employee knowingly follows a flawed procedure merely to cause damage."[80, p. 15] One can easily imagine a punished phlebotomist subsequently responding to a patient's complaint about bright lights by saying, "I have to turn the lights on. It's organization policy. You can blame them. Now hold still." There ought only be one goal of corporate punishment: to deter behavior that poses an unreasonable risk to corporate or client welfare. The phlebotomist came forward and reported the intentional error in the hope that the committee would become aware of and remedy latent system failures that encouraged the error. This is hardly the kind of behavior that should be deterred.

Assessing the Degree of Blamability for Process Violations

In his book, *Managing the Risks of Organizational Accidents,* James Reason offers an illuminating thought experiment originated by Neil Johnston and called the "substitution test" to assess blame. Reason suggests that an organization should:

> Substitute the (erring) individual … for someone else coming from the same domain of activity and possessing comparable qualifications and experience. Then ask the following question: "In light of how events unfolded and were perceived by those involved in real time, is it likely that this new individual would have behaved any differently?" If the answer is "probably not" then …. apportioning blame has no material role to play other than to obscure systemic deficiencies … A useful addition to the substitution test is to ask of the individual's peers: "Given the circumstances that prevailed at that time, could you be sure that you would not have committed the same or similar type of unsafe act?" If the answer again is "probably not," then blame is inappropriate.[81, p. 208]

Taking the example of an intentional process violation such as the phlebotomist's, the question arises: Would most phlebotomists have behaved as the one who actually committed the intentional error, and for the same reason? If so, the organization ought to be strongly inclined to reduce the penalty or refrain completely from imposing the penalty for the following reason: An organization ought not roundly penalize employees for intentional errors when a significant aspect of the employee's comprehension and justification of his or her violation points to a system failure that compromises patient care and prompts the violation.[82] "Blame" in such situations is borne collectively such that a committee member who insists the phlebotomist be penalized should also be asked to determine what portion of the blame the institution should itself bear for the system flaw that contributed to the phlebotomist's intentional violation.

Indeed, Reason's substitution test would be a provocative one to use with Dr. Anesthesiologist in the case study of Chapter 4. Would another anesthesiologist have made a similar error by thinking he turned the ventilator on and not realize it was still off because he had to leave his work station? Upon returning, would he then have failed to notice the ventilator was off for an indeterminate period of time because the alarms were suspended indefinitely? Would it be customary for the other health professionals in the operating room not to notice the absence of ventilation? Indeed, was the anesthesiology department somehow complicit in the disaster if the practice of deactivating the alarms on the anesthesia monitoring equipment was hospital wide?

I am arguing that unintentional harm-causing errors that occur in absence of process or standards violations ought merit no blame or punishment. Where there is a process violation such as the phlebotomist's infraction, the challenge for ascribing blame will be to determine whether 1) the error operator knew that his or her behavior constituted a process violation but did it anyway, or 2) was unaware of the process violation but should have known of it, or 3) was unaware of the process violation that was being committed because the institution failed to instruct him or her of the policy, or was negligent in monitoring the professional's clinical behavior. These issues and their implications can be folded into a discussion of reckless errors, to which I will now turn.

Reckless Errors

Reckless behavior by a health professional may be understood as an unallowable variation of process or professional behavior—and therefore a technical error in itself because it substantially deviates from the standard of care—that not only exposes another to an unreasonable amount of harm but that witnesses the health provider's disregard for the other's welfare.[83] Indeed, where the reckless perpetrator intends harm to occur, the action goes beyond the pale of ethics and becomes criminal.

Recklessness connotes an extreme breach of the fiduciary bond that anchors the professional-patient relationship, such that the patient who places his or her trust in the professional's discernment and skill is frankly betrayed. Penalizing the health professional in these instances should be predicated on the belief that punishment will have a deterrent effect, either on the professional's behavior or on the potentially reckless behavior of others.

Obviously, the easiest cases in which to determine recklessness are those wherein the health professional knew or should have known that his or her behavior unreasonably placed another in harm's way. There is little trouble in blaming and penalizing Dr. Jones (along with calling the institution to task) for not having more forcefully interceded to address Jones's alcoholism. Nevertheless, the penalty levied on Jones should also depend on whether or not the punishment would have a reasonable chance of returning Jones to the straight and narrow. Would he, for example, be willing to enter a recovery program for impaired physicians? Would he be willing to seek counseling and/or join Alcoholics Anonymous? If Jones scoffs at these suggestions or minimizes the errors with which he was involved, he is a poor candidate for any kind of rehabilitation and should probably (at least) be dismissed from the hospital.

Harder cases involve instances when the professional has no idea that his or her behavior is actually reckless, or when it is difficult to determine when a level of harm exposure has been reached that qualifies as reckless. Suppose, for instance, that the phlebotomist in the above case routinely labels tubes at the nurse's station, not because doing so relieves patients of the unpleasant glare of the hospital room's lights, but just because the phlebotomist feels more comfortable doing so. Furthermore, suppose the phlebotomist has no idea why the label-tubes-at-the-bedside rule is in place. Administrative personnel evaluating her conduct will have to consider whether or not the phlebotomist should have known the rule and its rationale. If both the rule and its rationale were known but were intentionally breached because of the phlebotomist's interest in her personal comfort, it would appear that blame and punishment are in order. If, on the other hand, the phlebotomist pleads ignorance to both the rule and its rationale, the organization should question whether the phlebotomist was properly informed and trained to comply with the hospital's rule. If the hospital believes that its own training efforts are inadequate, then one might argue that a system fault is largely responsible for the error and the phlebotomist ought only be properly trained in safe procedure. But if the hospital can justify its belief that its training efforts are adequate, then additional training coupled with punishment seems warranted.

Easy determinations of recklessness involve incidents where the healthcare professional both intends the reckless action as well as its outcome. Instances of malevolent damage or premeditated acts of harming; intentional acts of economic harm either to the organization or its clients; and acts of misrepresentation, blatant dishonesty, and false advertising all seem like categorical instances of perverse behavior that not only involve institutional but legal sanctions as well.[84]

Furthermore, some health professionals might display reckless *attitudes or beliefs* that an institution might want to address. In her fairly recent study of physicians in Great Britain, Marilyn Rosenthal quoted one as saying, "A patient asks for an antibiotic. You write something wrong or the chemist can't interpret your writing. If that happens often you'd worry, but it's acceptable once in a while because you're in a hurry. It's a basic mistake we're all prone to."[85, p. 20] This is a ghastly suggestion that, in its generosity toward physician error, makes the physician sound as though he's forgotten about obligations toward patients. Much more difficult determinations of recklessness occur when a professional intentionally violates a process standard for reasons ranging from the curious to the understandable. While his or her actions may appear reckless, their underlying intention was not. Thus, a professional can argue that latent system flaws disposed him to intentionally err; that the error was motivated by a well-meaning concern for the patient's comfort; that the error was perpetrated for years without any organizational intervention; or that he was working under immense stress and time pressures that the organization did little to minimize. The strength or weakness of each of these justifications necessarily look to the context of the situation itself and to the institutional atmosphere of patient safety, such that the error evaluators or blame assessors should be recruited on the basis of their good sense, experience, and inclination toward moral fairness.

Robert Lane notes how the evolution of scientific explanation will increasingly obscure the key factor that all acts of blame and punishment assume, viz., the agent's voluntariness.[86] Lane argues that scientific explanation is inherently causal and that the more we know about multifactorial causes, and especially about those causes of my behavior that I cannot control, the more my behavior seems determined. But the more it appears that I cannot exert control over my behavior, the less I am responsible for it and, therefore, the less I should be blamed or punished for it. Thus, suppose research on alcoholism convincingly shows that Dr. Jones's brain physiology made him immensely susceptible to alcoholism and that another aspect of his brain functioning and psychological formation dulled his self-awareness so much that he was unable to exercise reasonable insight into his addiction. How much should we blame and punish him then? How much can we impose punishments on persons for behaviors that they cannot reasonably control and for which social stigmas, and therefore disincentives, await those who seek help?

Lane further argues that the contemporary problem of free will is not an all-or-nothing dichotomy but rather, and consistent with my analysis of responsibility and blamability, a matter of degree. That is, some people can have more free will than others, "and therefore are more vulnerable to moral blame than those who have less free will."[87, p. 50] On this account, the better educated may be more blame-worthy than the poorly educated, because the inclination is to think that the former have more factual as well as moral insight and understanding of their actions, intentions, and the probable consequences.

While these are provocative issues, I will not elaborate on them here. Suffice it to say that the above analysis suggests the following blamability gradient in examining the conjunction of an unintended error with an unintended or intended process violation:

No blame/punishment:	* Unintended error not associated with an instittionally articulated process violation
	* Unintended error occurred in conjunction with a nonintentional process violation where the institution admits training was insufficient and/or latent system failures significantly facilitated the error
Modest (if any) blame/ punishment:	* Unintended error occurred in conjunction with an intentional, known process violation, but the professional can identify compelling mitigating circumstances (e.g., system flaws, patient-centered concerns) to explain the violation
Blame/punishment warranted:	* Unintended error occurred in conjunction with an uncomprehending process violation where the professional should have known the standard and no mitigating circumstances are present
	* Unintended error occurred in conjunction with an intentional process violation with no mitigaing circumstances present

Severe blame and punishment: * Intentional process violation with blatant disregard for the patient's welfare

                                              * Intent to harm the patient, irrespective of whether error or harm occurred

Ex Ante Versus Post Hoc Perspectives on Error Evaluation

In the anesthesiology case study that was discussed in Chapter 4, a very problematic blamability factor affecting Dr. Anesthesiologist was his failure to hear the pulse oxymeter alarm. This alarm occurs in the form of a beep whose tone gets lower as the oxygen saturation of the patient's blood decreases. While Dr. Anesthesiologist contended in his deposition that he had no idea that other alarms were programmed in a "suspend indefinite" mode and thus would not go off in any case, he himself may have turned the volume down on the pulse oxymeter so that it was inaudible. If he did, this process violation speaks to his blamability. If, on the other hand, the pulse oxymeter beep was audible but Dr. Anesthesiologist just did not notice it, then we can use James Reason's substitution test to assess the blamability of his nonvigilance.

This implies that individuals who are charged with deciding responsibility, blamability, and punishment need to possess objectivity and understanding about the phenomenon of harm-causing error as well as be sensitive toward the experience of error operators *before* an accident happens. As Richard Cook notes, system operators in the ex ante stage always work to produce desired results and are continuously implementing measures that forestall accidents.[88] Furthermore, given the immensely chaotic environment in which much of healthcare delivery occurs, system operators are probably multitasking, often in frequently stressful situations. To appreciate the circumstances of an error-resulting-in-harm trajectory, error evaluators must therefore empathically situate themselves in the "before accident" environment to appreciate how the error pathway developed and proceeded. Evaluating the error from the after-accident perspective "poisons the ability of after-accident observers to recreate the experience of the practitioners before the accident occurred."[89, p. 2] From the post hoc perspective, the errors that facilitated the harm will be obvious to anyone because the evaluator has no insight into the moment-to-moment experiential "thickness" of what the error operator had to confront and manage. An after-accident perspective inevitably witnesses certain "error moments" that stick out like sore thumbs because all the details that system operators were otherwise attending to are shorn away, leaving the crucial error moments in stark relief. It is easy to understand, then, how evaluators *who situate themselves in the post hoc perspective* might regard error operators as unforgiveably inept because the post-accident perspective encourages deleting the moment-by-moment cognitive static and materiel that the operator had to manage.[90]

Not only are the error trajectory and the events that facilitated it so patently obvious from the post hoc perspective, but sociologists observe that, "we cannot ignore the influence of personality, social class, and culture on the judges."[91, p. 55] As such, I want to explore the following hypotheses: 1) the tradition of blame and punishment as a reaction to error often reflects the organizational personality of healthcare training and delivery programs, especially as that personality is displayed by upper level management or leadership, and 2) compulsivity is a hallmark characteristic of that personality and explains in great part why error evaluators may be very disinclined to give up a blaming and punitive response to error.

Evaluating the Error Evaluators

In his entertaining and very wise book, *Emotional Vampires,* psychologist Albert Bernstein points out how work is the great passion of the compulsive personality: "It [work] is their pride, their joy, their obsession, their drug, the alpha and omega of their existence. It is their gift, and the cross they have to bear."[92, p. 184] He underlines the compulsive personality's trustworthiness, honesty, promise-keeping, valiant struggle to impose order on a chaotic universe, immense attention to detail, and never-ending dedication to excellence. Because compulsiveness is such a highly adaptive and socially valuable trait, its familiarity among supervisors, managers and, as we have seen, physicians should not be surprising. Gabbard says that, "it is probably accurate to assert that compulsive traits are present in the majority of those individuals who seek out medicine as a profession,"[93, p. 2926] and he cites studies wherein physicians overwhelmingly and proudly identify themselves as compulsive personalities. None of this should be surprising. Indeed, one suspects it is the rare patient who would not want his or her physician to be compulsive about patient care.

The connection of all this with blame and punishment occurs when we realize that the compulsive personality typically maintains a deeply held belief that pain, discipline, and delayed gratification are essential for maintaining an orderly and safe environment as well as to secure success and respect.[94] Pathological compulsives learn to be immensely fearful of doing anything wrong or wayward because failure shatters the delicate connection between their need to feel perfect and their fragile sense of self-esteem. Emphasizing the familiar psychological observation that our neuroses develop around what causes us the most anxiety and fear, mental health professionals assert that the compulsive's unhealthy behaviors, attitudes, and beliefs are a pathological reaction to his or her despised imperfections and occasional feelings of helplessness. In the compulsive's warped view of the world, success requires a stalwart and often painful diligence that repudiates all those tendencies and dispositions that smack of indifference, frivolity, inattentiveness, and lassitude.[95] Much more than most, the compulsive is extremely uncomfortable in the midst of those behaviors, which is why compulsives like to surround themselves with similarly compulsive persons. When failure occurs, the compulsive knows only to blame, as his or her comprehension scheme automatically connects failure with carelessness and irresponsibility and triggers his or her stereotypical response to error: inflicting pain.

Compulsives understand punishment as an intervention that improves or positively enables the self's moral character. In fact, punishment is a manifestation of the pathologically compulsive individual's self-loathing (or other-loathing) for failure to rise above imperfection.[96] Just as compulsives are enraged by their own errors and blame themselves excessively, they react similarly to the errors of others. The compulsive is convinced that punishment is what is owed the error operator—not even so much as a deterrence toward future commissions of error or as a vehicle for learning, but rather to appease the vengefulness of a relentlessly vigilant and cruel superego. As though the discomfort of his or her neurotic attention to detail is not pain enough, the compulsive knows only to punish him- or herself or others when things go wrong. Giving up that attitude and the false beliefs that support it may be immensely difficult for the compulsive, which is why these persons are not morally or psychologically qualified to assess responsibility and blame in instances of harm-causing error. Punishment is the default position for compulsives who confront error.

Blameless and Nonpunitive Environments and the Disclosure of Error

Ultimately, the development of a blameless and nonpunitive policy to manage error is a complementary but intermediate point in disclosing error to the harmed party because the policy itself says more about the conscience of the organization than it does about the practices of its personnel. It is obviously one thing to hold the erring professional organizationally blameless, but quite another to disclose his or her error to the harmed party so that the latter can make his or her determination regarding blame and reparations. What the blameless and nonpunitive policy will encourage is the reporting of error to the institution, not necessarily its disclosure to the harmed party.

Yet, organizational cultures or social atmospheres do indeed affect the values, beliefs, and attitudes of employees. In that respect, an approach to blame and punishment such as the one outlined above should send multiple messages of understanding, support, and moral objectivity regarding the commission of medical error. The first message is that error is remarkably democratic: No one is exempt or spared from its commission. Second, only in rare circumstances will such a policy indict an error operator's character or self. Rather, most interventions will focus on whatever behaviors need improvement. Also, if the model I have presented above is morally correct, many instances of error analysis will witness no blaming or penalizing intervention because the error will be shown to have been random, unintentional, and entirely typical of the kind of momentary lapses and mistakes that occur among all human beings. A third aspect of such a policy is its insistence on a thoughtful and responsible reaction to errors. Such a model assesses blame and adjudicates punishment in a reflective and responsible way, so that at least the error reporting, if not the error disclosure, aspect of error management occurs in a morally informed manner.

Last, one would like to think that all of this would ultimately encourage error operators to disclose their errors to the patients who are harmed. But if the professional, even after reporting the error to administration, still resists, one hopes that the organization will itself dispatch its moral responsibility to the harmed parties. One would like to think that an organization that is keen to act justly toward its staff is just as morally disposed toward its patients.

We reach a point in this analysis, then, where error disclosure, at least as it occurs in hospitals, involves a shared moral vision among its staff and their administration. Together, the two must maintain relatively similar beliefs and attitudes about the various moral elements that affect error reporting and disclosure as well as be able to summon the moral courage to report and disclose error appropriately. In the next section, we will examine how both administrative and clinical staff (who will be most personally affected by the commission of errors) might maintain a moral atmosphere that honors the harmed party's right to know about the occurrence of serious error.

Section 3 ■ Mindfulness

"Teaching" Ethics

Only recently have healthcare institutions begun to evince an interest in the psychological formation of health providers and examine the stressors and other factors that can compromise the delivery of compassionate and humanistic care. It is fair to say that for most of the twentieth century, it was assumed that if an individual gained admission to a healthcare training program, he or she ipso facto had the psychological stamina and constitution to withstand the rigors of the training and the workload. Beginning in the late 1970s, however, training institutions began to realize that they ought to prepare students to manage the occasional ethical problems that are inevitable in the delivery of healthcare, and so ethics instruction was gradually introduced to the curriculum.[97] As Jeffrey Burack and his colleagues note, however, "Contemporary medical ethics education has concerned itself with teaching either facts or moral reasoning procedures, but not with the motivational network of values, attitudes, and feelings that underlies moral behavior."[98, p. 49] A dominant theme of the contemporary literature on "teaching" humanistic medicine is that exploring this particular motivational network and its response to the psychological complexity and pressure of delivering healthcare goes a considerable way toward explaining why healthcare personnel sometimes seem less than caring and compassionate. While a stirring lecture on ethical behavior might have some utility, a far more powerful learning experience for the nursing or medical student will be his or her observations of what actually happens on the wards. Thus, my colleague William Branch recently declared, "My observations of students suggest that they perceive obstacles that undermine their care and compassion for patients as the chief moral problems that they face on the wards, less so hindrances that limit their ability to reason about ethical issues." [99, p. 505]

Although the tide may be shifting, there has long been a kind of Platonic conceit in bioethics instruction that if the student "knows" the right thing to do, he or she will do it. In fact, ample evidence suggests that confronting a moral dilemma or a lapse in professional behavior arouses considerable anxiety that health professionals often manage by avoidance. [100] Although the physician must always intervene in his or her patient's care according to the professional standard, he or she usually has considerable latitude in resisting what moral behavior frequently, if not most often, requires: finding the wherewithal to confront and process the moral issue through sustained dialogue and reflection with the principal parties and then implement responsible behavior.

Physicians are often criticized for resisting conversation in morally challenging situations, whether it be confronting a colleague who acts unprofessionally, discussing end-of-life issues with dying patients, or disclosing a medical error. In a pertinent paper published in 1999, Burack and his colleagues described how and why attending physicians often responded problematically to learner (in this case, residents' and medical students') behaviors that exhibited unprofessional attitudes toward patients. [101] These behaviors included showing disrespect for patients, cutting corners, and outright hostility or rudeness—behaviors that would go down as "unethical" on anyone's moral ledger. Burack's findings deserve a lengthy quotation:

> Attending physicians were rarely observed to respond to these problematic behaviors. When they did, they favored passive nonverbal gestures such as rigid posture, failing to smile, or remaining silent ... Attending physicians did not explicitly discuss attitudes, refer to moral or professional norms, "lay down the law," or call attention to their modeling, and rarely gave behavior-specific feedback. Reasons for not responding included lack of opportunity to observe interactions, sympathy for learner stress, and the unpleasantness, perceived ineffectiveness, and lack of professional reward for giving negative feedback ... They (i.e. attending physicians) tended to avoid, rationalize, or medicalize these behaviors, and to respond in ways that avoided moral language, did not address underlying attitudes, and left room for face-saving reinterpretations. [102, p. 49]

Avoidance of the unpleasant—which is linked with Meyer Gunther's axiomatic observation on the formation of narcissistic-like defenses in that "Anxiety must be avoided at all costs"—has to count as a fundamental reason for resistance to moral intervention. But if that is so, then a liability of such avoidance might well be the unintended fostering and development of uncaring, uncompassionate, narcissistic-like behaviors. How, then, might healthcare training programs implement strategies whereby mechanisms are in place to contain and process unprofessional behaviors so as to lessen the probability of their recurrence? As in the chapter on narcissism, I will postpone a discussion of error disclosure and revisit the precepts of empathy at some length. The reason is that overcoming narcissistically based defenses is key to encouraging the kind of morally appropriate feelings that health professionals should experience when they are tempted to offer the patient less than he or she is owed. An appreciation for how healthcare can do more to foster patient-centered sensibilities in emotionally taxing scenarios is an important element in the health professional's acceptance of a duty to disclose error—a duty that in certain instances might rank as the most anguishing moral responsibility a health professional can have.

Other Regard/Empathy Revisited

Whether it be the disclosure of a dreadful disease, a medical error, or a heart-to-heart conversation with a dying patient, the fundamental atmosphere and strategy of these conversations should be empathy, that is, the professional's appreciation and comprehension of how this experience is understood and felt by the other (e.g., as in "I wonder what it's like right now to be you, Mr. Jones.").[103] Because the empathic communicator understands the importance of his or her knowing what this experience *feels like and means to the listener*, the empathic health professional must have the ability to suspend his or her own framework of meaning so as to grasp the other's.[104] As we saw in previous chapters, the health professional who cannot get beyond his or her immediate discomfort of making a harm-causing error, and understand the event from the patient's point of view might not only bungle whatever conversation subsequently occurs but invite a lawsuit because the patient perceives the professional as uncaring. Obviously, the health professional who reverts to narcissistically based, emotionally insulating behaviors that favor disengagement when he or she feels psychologically threatened represents the antithesis of the empathic communicator. The empathic challenge is to transcend the comfort and familiarity of one's own world-view and tune into the world experience of another.[105] How, then, does a person develop the competencies to overcome the anxiety or resistance connected with entering the world experience of another? Because I will examine the mechanics of empathic conversations in considerable detail in the next chapter, what follows describes certain training and institutional strategies that lay the groundwork for the practice of empathy and the overcoming of narcissistic-like regressions in the face of emotional discomfort.

#1. Narrative competence. Physician-ethicist Rita Charon champions the idea of "narrative competence" wherein health professionals become more skillful at absorbing, interpreting, and responding to others' *stories*.[106] It is interesting to note how many health professionals, physicians in particular, have little time for or disdain the idea of listening to patients' stories. Whether they are pathologically impatient, unconvinced that stories contribute anything to the patient's clinical management, disdainful of the "soft" stuff of stories versus the hard objectivity of clinical data, or fearful that a careful listening to the patient's story would invite an anxiety-ridden departure from the psy-

chologically safe world of their own valuative beliefs and feelings, physicians are commonly indicted by patients for "not listening to me."[107]

A little reflection and a sizable literatures show, however, that clinical medicine is replete with stories and narratives, certain ones of which physicians adore. Grand rounds, morbidity and mortality conferences, banter in the physicians' dining rooms, and most professional committee work largely revolve around stories—indeed, they could not proceed without them.[108] Moreover, I have observed physicians virtually salivate as they elaborate on differential diagnoses in occult cases or on a particular interventional technique, as well as expect their medical students or residents to deliver comprehensive recitations of the patient's past and current medical history. What this suggests, then, is that there are certain kinds of stories that health professionals like, along with others they do not.

Narrative *incompetence* stems from a rigidly limited tolerance of what counts as salient in the patient's discourse. The essence of that limitation is the way the professional's beliefs and assumptions cause him or her to filter out and dismiss material whose content seems irrelevant to his or her epistemological (i.e., most probably the materialistic-reductionistic-Newtonian-germ theory) model of illness and disease.[109] One objective of achieving narrative competence, then, is for the professional to appreciate that the Western canon of physical science that so powerfully determines his or her comprehension of "clinical reality" is not universally shared and that his or her firm insistence that it be the regnant model for this understanding can be relationally disastrous. One remedy for this phenomenon is for the health professional to have a powerful, supportive, and appreciative encounter with valuative perspectives that offer a vastly different understanding of health, illness, medicine, life, and death from the professional's own.

In addition to encouraging literature seminars and reading groups so as to stimulate participants with imaginative experiences they might not otherwise have, Charon and similarly minded educators strongly endorse and implement narrative writing in their medical school curricula.[110] Here, the student is challenged to write a few pages on what is happening to the patient *from the patient's point of view*, or the student might be challenged to write about an emotionally uncomfortable situation he or she recently experienced and then share that material in a small discussion group. In the first instance, the student must deeply imagine what it is like to be the other, which might require the student to interview the patient to learn about the experience from the patient's viewpoint. In the second instance, the student is encouraged to visit and get nonjudgmentally in touch with his or her unpleasant or anxious feelings so as to explore their content and meaning. The point of nonjudgmental observations and descriptions of one's own feelings is to uproot whatever psychological censors might cause certain material to be deleted or withheld as unprofessional or inappropriate.[111] Because both of these exercises occur in groups in which participants are made to feel psychologically safe, individuals not only expand their own experiential horizons but often learn deep lessons about themselves and one another. The pedagogical objectives bent on overcoming narcissistic barriers to empathy are to select narrative material that is likely to expose persons to experiences they might otherwise not have and/or that trigger deeply felt personal reactions; to give individuals permission to have these feelings and to discuss them openly in a supportive environment; and to encourage reflection on those intensely personal, sometimes anguishing emotions in an atmosphere that is constructively critical, accepts an "imperfectionist" model of human behavior, and is deeply appreciative of our common humanity.[112] Because the development of narrative competence rests on the cusp of how learning about the other might lead to important self-revelations, we will discuss it more elaborately below. For now, let us only note that individuals who lead groups such as these should have considerable experience as facilitators, because discussions sometimes turn to material that can arouse deep feelings of inadequacy, anger, humiliation, frustration, and even self-destructiveness.

#2. The white coat and professional development. Here's an old joke: Two fellows are having a chat in heaven when an elderly but very distinguished-looking gentleman wearing a sterling white laboratory coat walks by. One asks the other, "Who's that?" The other responds, "Oh, that's God. He thinks he's a doctor."

A traditional medical school ceremony that occurs early in the student's experience is the donning of the white coat. Many institutions choreograph an elaborate white coat ceremony in which the student walks across a stage and is assisted by various deans and other high-ranking faculty in donning a white coat for the first time. While the physical dimensions of the coat itself are significant—the length of the coat reflects one's rank and authority, that is, medical students' coats are waist high, residents are usually mid-thigh, and a senior physician's coat will often be at or below the knee—the white color of the coat is taken to symbolize cleanliness, science (as in the "laboratory" coat), and healing. Add to this, as Delese Wear points out "the Western cultural meanings of whiteness—life, purity, innocence, superhuman power, goodness—and it is easy to see how the white coat became the favored garment for physicians."[113, p. 735]

Presumably, the white coat ceremony is intended to impress one and all with the altruistic values of medicine. Wear worries, however, that the ceremonial donning of the coat is the first ritualized, symbolic representation to the student of "care-giving hierarchies and spheres of practice, the social and economic privilege of physicians, and medicine's well-established practices (not unlike those of the law or the priesthood) in determining membership in the profession."[114, p. 735]

If the white coat ceremony is an unwitting but formal invitation to the narcissistic world we are exploring, and if a partial antidote to that tendency is the broadening of one's experiential horizons and narrative competence, then it might be well to have such newly garbed medical students rapidly exposed to a range of socially diverse contexts. Wear suggests that students be exposed to learning environments such as free clinics, reproductive services, food banks, drug and alcohol intervention programs, domestic violence shelters, adult day care centers, rape crisis centers, or hospices. Therein, students would meet, treat, and learn from a wide swath of humanity—many of whom the student might find forbidding or repulsive. But therein lies the value of ascribing meaning to the white coat by juxtaposing students' early idealism and natural empathy with a kind of human suffering and misery that many of these students could not begin to imagine. Again, these exposures should be intellectually and emotionally processed in groups, for example, as Charon does in her narrative writing classes. Because members of the group openly share and explore their own and others' insights and feelings, they cannot help but be affected in ways that a formal lecture could barely touch.

#3. Role modeling. Like most professional preparations, learning the interventional facets of medicine best occurs by observation, then doing, then receiving feedback, then repeated doing with more feedback.[115] Recalling our previous discussion about the creation of a moral atmosphere, it is crucial for learners to observe role models who, by definition, model morally ideal behaviors. It would be helpful to have more empirical data on the psychological formation of such role model physicians, such as the study that Mohammedreza Hojat and his colleagues conducted on comparing personality profiles of internal medicine residents with physicians whom the residents identified as role models.[116] Hojat's findings suggest that these role models accommodated the characterization of the "healthy narcissist" as discussed in Chapter 3 to a remarkable degree. Using the revised NEO Personality Inventory and comparing 188 role model physicians with 104 internal medicine house officers, Hojat found that role model physicians were more likely to be co-operative, more eager to face challenges and contribute to solving problems, had higher self-esteem, were dominant, forceful, and exerted more energy and yet were less prone to anger, craved sensation less (i.e., they had lower sensation-seeking scores), were less cynical, better able to control their impulses, and better able to cope with adversity.[117] In comparison with the residents and a representative sample of the adult U.S. population, Hojat's role model physicians had lower anxiety, anger, depression, self-consciousness, impulsivity, and vulnerability scores. Despite the stressors of practicing medicine, these role-model physicians presented a remarkable picture of vibrant, emotionally healthy human beings.

One wonders whether the vitality and interest these physicians exhibited in their work weren't as influential in prompting residents to identify them as role models as the skills they displayed in treating patients. In a study by Bill Branch and his colleagues that sought to answer the question, "What might be done in the patient's presence to improve and teach the human dimensions of care?" respondents identified role modeling as the *sole* teaching method.[118] Exemplary physician-teachers were ones who:

- Asked permission to enter the patient's room
- Ensured privacy by pulling curtains
- Paid attention when the patient was short of breath or in pain
- Physically touched the patient
- Sat down beside the patient during rounds
- Personally adjusted the patient's pillows and bedspreads
- Replaced trays
- Asked about the patient's personal life and his or her family
- Measured the patient's pulse during a bedside interview—thus initiating physical touch as well as implementing a symbolic, caring gesture

Branch noted that role models and students usually had a discussion prior to entering the patient's room as to how the teacher would address the patient's issues, such as the patient's unhappiness with hospital routine, overall discomfort, refusal to agree to diagnostic studies, or need for informed consent. Similarly, role models processed with learners what occurred immediately after a clinical encounter so as to "promote understanding of the observed behavior and help solidify learning."[119, p. 1071] Obviously, a key element in these role-modeling exercises is for students to observe how model professionals disclose bad news. As we will note in the next chapter about the mechanics of error disclosure, an explicit set of communication strategies is now recognized that fosters the kind of empathic communications that identifies role models as role models.

All of this learning—whether it be Charon's interest in narrative competence, clinical observations and experiences among socio-economically marginalized populations, or Branch's descriptions of role model physicians—occurs in environments of openness, personal safety, support, and respect. Learners need to feel respected if they are to respect others. They need to be encouraged to feel *and accept* their own real feelings, however raw, uncomfortable, and scarred they might be, if they are to respect the feelings of others. And they need to feel that the exploration of the humanistic care of patients is as credible and important a component of their education as anatomy, physiology, and pharmacology. Moreover, they should be impressed with the idea that much of humanistic medicine is skill-based—that it is subserved by a body of knowledge and techniques that can be practiced and learned.[120] And one of the most important of the empathic techniques to learn, especially in disclosing medical error, is how to use and appreciate silence.

#4. *Practicing silence and attentive listening*. The health professional who is open to be other-regarding must be other-respecting, and one of the most basic expressions of respect for the other is a concentrated silence that attends to the other's every word, every sigh, every pause, every vocal inflection, and every facial nuance and physical gesture. Just as the participants in Charon's literature seminars must silence their own belief systems to grasp the other's and to respectfully attend to their peers, so the communicator bent on empathy must respect the other through keenly attentive listening, which requires silence.

Like radio announcers, health professionals are frequently not good with silence. Perhaps because they wrongly understand silence as wasteful inactivity, many health professionals respond to soundlessness by feeling anxious, bewildered, overwhelmed, ignorant, or inadequate.[121] Because these are uncomfortable feelings, health professionals have a marked but understandable inclination to fill up acoustical space with the sound of their voice, which tends to soothe their anxieties. What professionals neglect to consider is how staying their own impulse to react can therapeutically affect the patient, who, if he or she feels respectfully heard by an authority figure, may well feel like the center of the universe. Not surprisingly, patients who find themselves center-stage and bathed in a spotlight of respect will often open up to their caretakers, regard the clinical relationship as more trusting and therapeutic, and possibly experience better outcomes. In disclosing medical error, the communicator who speaks briefly and who listens respectfully will have a markedly more favorable effect on the patient—no matter how wretched the conversation becomes—than the one who is constantly succumbing to the urge to clarify, interpret, explain, and dominate the conversation.[122]

If other-regard requires a respect that is often best conveyed by a respectful silence, health providers should also practice attentive listening. He or she might resolve, for example, not to interrupt the patient except with an occasional "uh-huh" or "tell me more about that" for the first two minutes of conversation (which some professionals will find exceedingly difficult). Of keen importance during such an exercise is for the professional not only to be focused on the patient's narrative but to silence his or her "inner voices" and allow him- or herself to be absorbed by the moment.[123] Not only is the incessant pager and cell phone the bane of respectful attention, but health professionals become so used to working at a frenetic pace that they forget what calmness and unstructured time feels like. Allowing themselves to simply "be" in the moment and do nothing except absorb the patient's words and silences can feel unstructured, unfamiliar, and uncomfortable. Glen Gabbard wrote about a physician couple who forced themselves to get away from their extremely hectic practices and finally take their long-promised vacation in the Bahamas. He described how, "The first morning on the beach was quite disconcerting, because they had no schedule to follow. Their response was to begin scheduling activities to structure the week. Every time they walked along the beach, they experienced vague feelings about not 'doing something.' Throughout the week they had to remind themselves repeatedly that doing nothing was a legitimate way to spend a vacation."[124, pp. 32–33] In her book, *The Scalpel's Edge*, Pearl Katz described a head of surgery who purposely arranged his administrative schedule so he would be constantly interrupted. He had gotten so used to being distracted and to filling every second of his conscious activity with "doing something" that he felt oddly uncomfortable when moments of empty time occurred.[125]

Some professionals, especially the compulsive ones, must learn to silence the internal, mental talk that they incessantly hear. The problem is that for so many of them, the mental clamor they hear inside their skulls becomes so familiar that they fail to notice how it causes them to read and write in the patient's medical notes rather than look at and listen to the patient during an interview; how the pressure to be productive causes them to frequently interrupt the patient's discourse; how their constant rush to see the next patient signals a devaluation of whomever they are with; and how such inattentiveness and impatience gradually become fixtures of their personality.[126]

Obviously, relaxation and meditative practices can be powerful aids in diminishing these feelings and their associated behaviors, but it is often the case that achieving an attentive silence resonates with cultivating one's humility. Buddha deemed humility the first of his noble truths, and psychiatrist Mark Epstein, in his wonderful book *thoughts without a thinker*, argues that the essence of Buddhism consists in its assisting humankind to overcome its natural tendency toward narcissistic self-preoccupation.[127]

Although more will be said about Epstein's book in the last chapter, consider how the authentically humble self recognizes and accepts human finitude and how silence is a remarkably fitting response to that realization. Whereas the arrogant self—and in its most exaggerated pathological form, the evil self—recognizes and respects no limits and seeks to overwhelm the world, the humble self understands his or her immensely limited capacity to know, to affect others, and to control his or her personal destiny as well as the destinies of others.[128] People interested in the phenomenon of narcissism might find it provocative to learn that four questions the Buddha would never entertain were whether:

- The world is eternal, or not, or both, or neither
- The world is finite (in space), or infinite, or both, or neither
- An enlightened being exists after death, or does not, or both, or neither
- The soul is identical with the body or different from it[129]

Interestingly, and perhaps serving as a testimony to the intellectual narcissism of the West, these are the very questions that have preoccupied Western philosophy, science, and religion since the ancient Greeks.

The humble, narcissistic-avoiding health professional is likely to respect otherness because of his or her basic respect for human dignity and equality; is likely to pay more attention to the patient because of a belief that the patient's discourse can hold significant insights and clues that contribute toward a more accurate diagnosis and productive course of treatment; and is likely to think of the professional-patient interrelationship as a vitalizing therapeutic tool, rather than esteem his or her clinical acumen as the sole variable that will effect the patient's recovery.[130] By humbling and silencing my "self," I enable others to guide and inform what I do. In the midst of a harried workload and feeling overwhelmed with responsibility, the health professional might remember the story wherein the Buddha was asked what he is, to which he responded with a precious double-entendre, "I am awake."[131]

#5. Being awake and mindfulness. It is worth noting how the above paragraphs segued from factors encouraging empathic environments to factors bearing on one's interiority, that is, his or her beliefs, feelings, values, and attitudes. While a pictorial representation of empathy might posit a ray of attention that proceeds from the health professional to the patient, that ray obviously originates from the professional. As Dennis Novack and his colleagues observed, "However well physicians have learned the science of medicine, they use themselves to practice its art."[132, p.502] The following paragraphs explore this use of the self by discussing strategies whereby an empathic self can be cultivated through its own self-awareness and mindfulness. The empathic ray of attention must be willed by the self who, in practicing empathy, must manage his or her self-interest. In the words of Michael and Abigail Lipson, "[H]ow we hamper ourselves through a faulty kind of self-knowledge (dense with self-consciousness) must itself be known in its phenomenological course. Our deficiencies in attentional capacity lead to a host of ailments."[133, p. 21]

We can think of mindfulness as a person's becoming more insightful about the nature of his or her physical and mental processes during ordinary, everyday tasks. Mindfulness in healthcare is a practice that "extends beyond examining the affective domains and involves critical reflection on action, tacit personal knowledge, and values in all realms of clinical practice, teaching, and research."[134, p. 838] Ronald Epstein suggested that a key variable that affects the nature and degree of one's mindfulness is curiosity about one's *real* self. Here we must recall Masterson's contrast of the real and false selves. Whereas the real self "does not block feelings or deaden the impact of emotions,"[135, p. 42] the motives of the false self "are not to deal with reality tasks but to implement defensive fantasies ... The purpose of the false self is not adaptive but defensive, it protects against painful feelings."[136, p. 23] The medical narcissist's self-curiosity is surely focused on the false self, which has been carefully polished and cultivated over the years and which offers both fascination and protection. To the unhealthy narcissist's way of thinking, the false self represents a triumph over the real, feeling self whose imperfections, mistakes, clumsiness, shortcomings, fears, and insecurities are repudiated and disowned. The healthy narcissist, on the other hand, not only accepts his or her limitations and humanness with grace and maturity, but wants to explore them more deeply. His or her curiosity will be especially directed toward his or her frustrations and anger, which are common responses to organizational complexity, errors, unanticipated outcomes, human suffering, and death.

The mindful individual will be curious about the architecture of his or her frustrations and anger, such as:

- What sorts of patients elicit an angry reaction in me?
- What work situations usually make me angry and why?
- What are my usual responses to my own anger and the anger of others (e.g., do I overreact, placate, blame others, suppress my feelings, become super-reasonable)?
- What are the underlying feelings when I become angry (e.g., feeling rejected, humiliated, unworthy)?
- Where did I learn my responses to anger?[137, p. 504]

But the nonmindful, unhealthily narcissistic self allows no place for such curiosity because he or she *needs anger as a primary defense.* The unhealthy narcissist's exploration of his or her anger, fears, insecurities, or anxieties would require a confrontation with the real self hiding behind that emotional armor. The behaviorist Marsha Linehan remarked how many persons are "phobic" toward their own emotions, especially the ones they repeatedly experience and are most identified with because they sense that investigating those aspects of their selves would be too painful.[138, p. 194] That resistance explains why pathological narcissists are extremely poor self-monitors and why they resist counseling and therapy. While advanced narcissists can be too far gone in their pathology to be mindful, mechanisms are nevertheless available for "the narcissist in us all" to undertake a supportive and skillfully guided exploration in mindfulness.

#6. Mindfulness and Balint groups. One of the more interesting approaches to assisting health professionals, especially physicians, to develop mindfulness are Balint groups. Named after the English-Hungarian psychoanalyst Michael Balint, these groups concentrate on "a synthesis of cognitive and affective processing that leads the physician to a more precise, empathic and practical understanding of doctor/patient interactions and difficult patients."[139, p. 4] The group is usually comprised of eight to ten (usually family practice or internal medicine) physicians who meet once weekly for about an hour. Groups typically last for a few years although some have continued for well over a decade. Invariably, the focus of the meeting is a problematic case, presented by one of the participants. The discussion is facilitated by a skilled, group leader usually trained in mental health.

The group does not criticize the presenter's handling of the case, nor does the group zero in on eliciting disclosures about the presenter's personal self, although self-revelatory comments are common. The group functions neither as physician therapy nor didactic seminar. It does not attempt to break down the presenter's defenses as he or she recites and analyzes the case, nor does the group consider the physician's personal difficulties in relation to colleagues, family, or personal psychological history.[140] Rather, its focus is always on the professionalism of the physician-patient relationship. That focus, however, is largely on the physician-presenter's emotional response to the patient because that response, the kind of patient who triggers it, and the relational lumps and bumps that are described constitute the core of the group's discussion. Typical questions that punctuate group conversations are, "What was the patient's actual reason for coming that day?" "How did you feel when you saw the patient's name on your list?" "What kinds of thoughts and feelings did you have?"[141, p. 5]

The skill of the group leader is crucial for a number of reasons. He or she must keep the conversation contained within the physician-patient relationship; discourage over-interrogation of the presenter; maintain an air of safety and spontaneity; manage discussions that can include the participants' description of their thoughts and feelings; protect group members from hurtful criticisms or invasions of their privacy; and represent the absent patient if the discussion becomes lopsided in protecting the physician-presenter's emotional equanimity.[142]

Frank Dornfest, a leader of the Balint movement in the United States, describes the overall goals for Balint groups in a way that speaks directly to empathy. Dornfest remarks that in the group discussion process, members learn to suspend their own intruding perceptions and emotional reactions at the root of their habitual responses or blind spots.[143] Interestingly, when physicians begin to relate their cases, they often behave like the patient while the listeners behave like the physician. But because the group is concerned with understanding what each party brings to the relationship and how each affects the other, the group inevitably explores what it might have felt like to be the patient, how the patient might have transferred painful or troublesome psychic material to the physician, and how the physician's counter-transferential reaction influenced what subsequently occurred.[144] Because the atmosphere of the group is safe and supportive and discussions favor a reflective, exploratory, and spontaneous approach, group members gradually begin to consciously explore and discuss what might have been largely unconscious and repressed feelings, attitudes, values, and beliefs. The anticipated end-product of these reflections is that the physician learns how to use the therapeutic relationship successfully as well as learns to understand patient interactions in ways that lead to less frustration, professional unhappiness, and burnout.

#7. Other supportive/curricular groups. Some organizations have instituted periodic group discussions to provide psychological support, foster education, remediate organizational conflict, and enhance the development of empathy. In her study of the evolution of nursing expertise, Patricia Benner found that these groups—especially ones that include an interdisciplinary mix of professionals wherein each participant felt he or she would be heard and respected, and wherein professional discouragements, embarrassments, and errors could be discussed—were highly conducive to professional growth.[145]

These groups can be molded around "meaningful experience discussions," wherein presenters offer stories about powerful teachers, patients, critical incidents, and other learning moments in their lives that greatly influenced their professional and personal formations. Or a group experience might revolve around sharing clinical effectiveness strategies that especially involve difficult patients or emotionally painful situations. It is common to witness veteran health professionals, especially ones with a reputation for caring and compassion, becoming quite emotional in telling these stories, which, in turn, permits other group members to experience their feelings deeply.[146]

A provocative exercise that sometimes becomes the core focus of a group is "family of origin" discussions. Here, participants construct personal genograms or family trees that depict relationships bearing on familial roles, expectations, conflicts, and familial strengths and weakness. Novack and his colleagues describe how:

> Certain interaction patterns may be passed from generation to generation. Examples are attitudes and behaviors concerning intimacy, anger, and conflict resolution. One learns first from one's family about the nature, benefits, and pitfalls of caring, about the roles of the caregiver, about the balance of giving and receiving, about the communicative aspects of illness, and about how to respond to distress … Patients may remind physicians of family members with similar problems or behavioral patterns. Unrecognized identification of patients with family members can elicit feelings including fears of harming the patient, of inadequacy, of loss of control, and of addressing certain difficult topics. [147, p. 503]

Of course, curricular exercises that include interpersonal skills training wherein participants are videotaped with actual or simulated patients and then are critiqued are invaluable. It is amazing what a patient's anxious questions such as, "Doc, what's going on with me? No one's talking to me. Am I dying?" can elicit from a well-meaning but empathically untrained student or professional. As we will see in the next chapter, supportive and comforting responses are available and learnable for these kinds of situations such that anyone can become a reasonably adept bad news communicator.

Managing Resistance to Error Disclosure

Advanced or considerably pathological medical narcissists suffer from a very mistaken belief: that authentic fulfillment occurs only if they replace their real, imperfect self with an ideal, fantasized self. Even low-level narcissists might strive, with varying degrees of energy, to achieve or merge with that idealized self, while highest-level narcissists categorically believe they *are* that ideal self.[148] The farther along one's narcissism, the more it will be that perceived injuries to the ideal self will "display a vacillation between rage, shame, and feelings of emptiness."[149, p. 408] While integral to the narcissistic formation, beliefs that sustain a "perfection fantasy" are not only unrealistic but explain the narcissistic-like regressions that are typical of many health professionals' behaviors when things go wrong and the perfection fantasy is assaulted.

Using the group models described above, professionals would do well to focus their mindfulness on medical errors. Novack suggests that these group discussions revolve around five key questions:

- What was the nature of my mistake?
- What are my beliefs about the mistake?
- What emotions did I experience in the aftermath of the mistake?
- How did I cope with the mistake?
- What changes did I make in my practice as a result of the mistake?[150]

In these kinds of discussions, it is probably advisable not only to have trained facilitators, but also professionals wizened about the systemic nature of error. The penchant of many professionals is to target a single individual as the blameworthy party. This strategy is psychologically soothing on a number of grounds: It offers a quick, and therefore comforting, solution to a nasty problem; it relieves the anxious discomfort connected with having to conduct what could be a tedious, time-consuming investigation; it is a relief to the finger pointer to indict someone else as the blameworthy party; it helps the finger pointer to maintain a personal belief in his or her own perfection; it encourages the false but comforting belief that the root cause of the error has indeed been identified; it perpetuates the false belief that once the error operator can remediate whatever deficiency led to the error, perfection is still attainable; and by quickly dispatching the problem, it alleviates the guilt that professionals can feel in having betrayed the patient through error.

Novack and his colleagues not only identify the perfection fantasy as the root cause of these reactions, but list the unproductive sequelae of the perfection fantasy when a serious error occurs, such as feelings of excessive guilt and shame, ordering excessive tests to avoid future mistakes, inappropriately treating future patients based on over-generalizing from a mistake, mistakenly defining an errorless adverse outcome as due to error, refusing to discuss mistakes with others, and offering misleading information to patients or their families.[151]

Repeated discussion and empathic reflection on error would offer health profession-als a more professionally informed perspective and encourage processing the error in an organizationally healthy way. What is clear from Novack's observations and categori-cally supportive of one of the fundamental contentions of this book is that aversion to error acknowledgment and disclosure is robust among many health professionals because it is systemically supported by an historically ingrained set of beliefs, values, and attitudes deriving from the perfection fantasy. Consequently, the kinds of group discussions and exercises described above, where fallibilities and limitations are ack-nowledged as human and inevitable, where crushing feelings of inadequacy are thera-peutically processed, and where the health professional's self is supportively explored, should facilitate improved caregiving and reasonably comprehensive explanations of harm-causing error to the affected parties.

Managing Rationalizations of Error

Rationalizing a serious harm-causing medical error so as to conceal it or to justify a mis-leading representation of it to the affected parties can be significantly averted by organi-zational efforts that are keen to determine what actually occurred. Because the essential objective of the rationalization is to distort reality or slant it in a way favorable to the error operators, various institutional processes, especially as part of the organization's continuous quality improvement and risk management efforts, can and doubtlessly do counteract the rationalizing phenomenon.

For example, Martin Smith and Heidi Forster encourage the identification of latent system failures, that is, the disasters waiting to happen; standardizing procedures so as to avert an unreasonable degree of process variation; establishing clinical safeguards and monitoring how well they are followed and how effective they are; and understanding errors as an important dimension of utilization review and quality assurance operations. They also urge the codification of written protocols for managing errors; developing studies and writing projects on how to confront errors with a view toward publishing those accounts; and adopting institutional policies on how to disclose error that include how to proceed when an error operator refuses to disclose.[152]

In her article on moral rationalization that was discussed in Chapter 2, Jo-Ann Tsang suggested a "victim-centered" approach to combat rationalization, whereby an organi-zation can use "situational manipulation" to make it more difficult to rationalize. The essence of this approach is that because rationalizers seek to avoid and minimize either the error or the harm it causes, efforts that counteract avoidance and minimization will make the rationalizer's success less probable.[153]

To combat avoidance, Tsang suggests that persons who have admitted harming oth-ers tell their stories so that potential rationalizers can have their motivations "defied" as well as understand disclosure as an organizationally anticipated reaction to harm-causing error. Also, the "victimizer" might receive maximum feedback on the harm that was done, so that his or her inclination toward minimization is countered. A third strategy is to conduct discussion groups where would-be avoiders of error disclosure are criticized for their morally inappropriate behavior, while a fourth strategy is simply to identify and refute the error perpetrator's rationalizations by showing their real motivation.[154]

Perhaps the most direct way to combat error minimization is for the error operators to hear from the parties harmed by the error. Because the former will often expend considerable mental effort to convince themselves that the damage done was regrettable but dismissable, feedback from the aggrieved party often serves as a strong countermeasure.[155] As the case study and chapter on forgiveness illustrated, harmed parties tend to perseverate on the gravity of the error if the error operators make no attempt to acknowledge the error and apologize. So, in addition to educating staff on the literature as to what harmed parties want to hear in the event of error, another strategy a morally courageous hospital might consider is inviting a harmed party to speak to the staff about how he or she was affected by the error. Giving voice to victims of medical error changes their identity from a bad outcome statistic into a human being who was frankly wronged by the system. That humanization tends to facilitate an empathic response from the wrongdoers and thus disappoint the very objective that minimization hopes to achieve. Because it occurs in an organizational setting that is intent on emphasizing its patient-centered sensibilities and obligations, there is a good chance that these kind of public revelations might also facilitate the process of expiation and forgiveness.

Conclusion

This third section of the chapter is based on the premise that the mindful health professional will, in the event of a harm-causing medical error, be keenly aware of how his or her motivations, behaviors, attitudes, values, and beliefs affect error communication.

"Transparency" has lately become a popular word in the parlance of ethics.[156] Connoting a keenness and thoroughness of moral insight and understanding, transparency for the health professional who is involved in error ultimately results in a painful confrontation with his or her fallibility and a farewell to those perfectionistic fantasies that, for however long, offered immense psychological comfort, even intoxication. Of course, a confrontation with and acceptance of the real, imperfect self is not enough to ensure morally appropriate behavior in the instance of harm-causing error. But the health professional who can resonate with the patient's experience is surely in a better position to disclose error than the one who is so "dense with self-consciousness" that the other's experience is entirely removed from his or her awareness. Many health professionals resist mindfulness in the event of medical errors perhaps because they already know that patients are owed the truth and nothing less. One hopes that the above exercises and strategies will assist professionals to do the right thing when doing the right thing is dreadfully difficult.

References

1. Albert, Tanya. Physicians feel double-digit pain as liability rates continue to rise. *Amednews.com*, Nov. 10, 2003; Kazel, Robert. AMA report spotlights rising insurance premiums. *Amednews.com*, Sept. 15, 2003; Plummer, Alan. Medical liability in Georgia: the crisis is now. *Momentum*, Winter, 2003, available at http://www.emory.edu/WHSC/HSNEWS/PUB?Momentum/Winter03/onpoint.html.

2. Meyers, Susan Laccetti. Malpractice premiums on a rocket ride. *Atlanta Journal Constitution*, Sunday, August 11, 2002, Q1 and Q8.

3. Meyers, 2002.

4. Meyers, 2002; Plummer, 2003.

5. Albert, Tanya. Revisiting the crisis in Nevada: tort reform in need of reform. *Amednews.com*, Feb. 23, 2004.

6. King, Joseph H. *The Law of Medical Malpractice in a Nutshell*, 2nd edition. St. Paul, MN: West Publishing Company, 1986, p. 289.

7. Council on Ethical and Judicial Affairs. *Code of Medical Ethics: Current Opinions with Annotations*. 2002–2003 Edition. Chicago,IL: AMA Press, 2002.

8. Plummer, 2003.

9. Albert, Tanya. Tort reform wouldn't dent health spending—CBO report. *Amednews.com*, Feb. 23, 2004.

10. Hunter, J. Robert. Consumer viewpoint on the turmoil in the medical malpractice market. *Law and Bioethics Report* (Institute for Bioethics, Health Policy, and Law at the Louisville School of Medicine). 3(1):5–7, 2003.

11. Ouzts, Elizabeth. Cap on malpractice awards will solve nothing. *News & Record*, Sunday Edition, Sept. 28, 2003, H3, Greensboro, N.C.

12. McClellan, Frank M. Tort reform for medical malpractice cases: Stories vs. statistics. *Law and Bioethics Report* (Institute for Bioethics, Health Policy, and Law at the Louisville School of Medicine). 3(1):7–9, 2003.

13. Abraham, Kenneth S., and Weiler, Paul C. "Enterprise medical liability and the evolution of the American healthcare system." *Harvard Law Review*. 108(4): 381–436, 1994.

14. King, 1986.

15. King, 1986.

16. Abraham and Weiler, 1994.

17. Abraham and Weiler, 1994.

18. Abraham and Weiler, 1994.

19. Abraham and Weiler, 1994.

20. King, 1986.

21. Abraham and Weiler, 1994.

22. Abraham and Weiler, 1994.

23. Abraham and Weiler, 1994.

24. Abraham and Weiler, 1994.

25. Leape, Lucien L. "Error in medicine." *JAMA.* 272(23):1851–1857, 1994.

26. Sparger v. Worley Hosp., Inc., 547 S.W.2d 582.b.

27. Abraham and Weiler, 1994.

28. Abraham and Weiler, 1994.

29. Abraham and Weiler, 1994.

30. Abraham and Weiler, 1994.

31. Hickson, Gerald B.; Federspiel, C. F.; Pichert, J. W.; Miller, C. S.; Gauld-Jaeger J.; Bost, P. "Patient complaints and malpractice risk." *JAMA.* 287(22):2951–2957, 2002.

32. Abraham and Weiler, 1994.

33. Albert, Feb. 23, 2004.

34. Abraham and Weiler, 1994.

35. Studdert, David M., and Brennan, Troyen A. "Toward a workable model of 'no-fault' compensation for medical injury in the United States." *American Journal of Law & Medicine.* 27:225–252, 2001.

36. Studdert and Brennan, 2001.

37. Studdert and Brennan, 2001.

38. Bovbjerg, Randall, and Sloan, Frank A. "No-fault for medical injury: Theory and evidence." *University of Cincinnati Law Review.* 67(3):53–123, 1998.

39. Bovbjerg and Sloan, 1998.

40. Bovbjerg and Sloan, 1998.

41. Bovbjerg and Sloan, 1998.

42. Brennan, Troyen A.; Hebert, Liesi E.; Laird, Nan M.; Lawthers, Ann; Thorpe, Kenneth E.; Leape, Lucian L.; Localio, Russell A.; Lipsitz, Stuart R.; Newhouse Joseph P.; Weiler, Paul C.; Hiatt, Howard H. "Hospital characteristics associated with adverse events and substandard care." *JAMA.* 265(24): 3265–3269, 1991.

43. Bovbjerg and Sloan, 1998.

44. Bovbjerg and Sloan, 1998.

45. Bovbjerg and Sloan, 1998.

46. Bovbjerg and Sloan, 1998.

47. Bovbjerg and Sloan, 1998.

48. Bovbjerg and Sloan, 1998.

49. Bovbjerg and Sloan, 1998.

50. Bovbjerg and Sloan, 1998.

51. Bovbjerg and Sloan, 1998.

52. Bovbjerg and Sloan, 1998.

53. Bovbjerg and Sloan, 1998.

54. Bovbjerg and Sloan, 1998.

55. Bovbjerg and Sloan, 1998.

56. Bovbjerg and Sloan, 1998.

57. Bovbjerg and Sloan, 1998.

58. Studdert and Brennan, 2001; Bovbjerg and Sloan, 1998.

59. Studdert and Brennan, 2001.

60. Leape, 1994; also see Ladd, John. "Bhopal: An essay on moral responsibility and civic virtue." *Journal of Social Philosophy.* Spring:73–91, 1991; Lane, Robert E. "Moral blame and causal explanation." *Journal of Applied Philosophy.* 17(1):45–58, 2000.

61. Reason, James. *Managing the Risks of Organizational Accidents.* Aldershot, UK: Ashgate, 1997; Cook, Richard. How complex systems fail: being a short treatise on the nature of failure; how failure is evaluated; how failure is attributed to proximate cause; and the resulting new understanding of patient safety. University of Chicago: Chicago, IL, 1998. Available from ri-cook@uchicago.edu.

62. Cook, Richard, and Woods, David. "Operating at the sharp end: The complexity of human error." In *Human Errors in Medicine,* ed. Bogner, Marilyn Sue, Hillsdale, N.J.: Lawrence Erlbaum Associates, 1994, pp. 255–310.

63. Wolf, Zane Robinson. *Medication Errors: The Nursing Experience.* Albany, N.Y.: Delmar Publishers, 1994.

64. Kohn, Linda T.; Corrigan, Janet M.; and Donaldson, Molla S. *To Err Is Human: Building a Safer Health System.* Washington, DC: National Academy Press, 2000; also see Hill, Charlene D. Joint Commission commends patient safety and quality improvement act. Press release by the Joint Commission, Oakbrook Terrace, IL, June 7, 2002 (contact: chill@jcaho.org).

65. Marx, David. Patient safety and the "Just Culture"; a primer for healthcare executives. New York: Columbia University, 2001. (A manuscript prepared by David Marx, JD, for Columbia University under a grant provided by the National Heart, Lung, and Blood Institute.)

66. Reason, 1997.

67. Feinberg, Joel. *Harm to Others: The Moral Limits of the Criminal Law.* New York: Oxford University Press, 1984.

68. Lane, 2000; Ladd, 1991; Feinberg, 1984.

69. Feinberg, 1984.

70. Banja, J. "When harms become wrongs: Some comments on the moral language of oppression and the limitations of moral theory." *Journal of Disability Policy Studies.* 12(2):79–86, 2001.

71. Banja, 2001.

72. Govier, Trudy. *Forgiveness and Revenge.* London: Routledge, 2002.

73. Govier, 2002.

74. Marx, 2001.

75. Lane, 2000; Marx, 2001.

76. See, for example, the American Society for Healthcare Risk Management's Code of Professional Ethics and Conduct. Available at http://www.ashrm.org.

77. Marx, 2001; Reason, 1997.

78. Marx, 2001.

79. Marx, 2001.

80. Marx, 2001.

81. Reason, 1997.

82. Reason, 1997; Ladd, 1991.

83. Marx, 2001.

84. Marx, 2001.

85. Rosenthal, Marilyn. *The Incompetent Doctor: Behind Closed Doors.* Berkshire, UK: Open University Press, 1995.

86. Lane, 2000.

87. Lane, 2000.

88. Cook, 1998.

89. Cook, 1998.

90. Cook, 1998.

91. Lane, 2000.

92. Bernstein, Albert J. *Emotional Vampires: Dealing with People Who Drain You Dry.* New York: McGraw Hill, 2001.

93. Gabbard, Glen O. "The role of compulsiveness in the normal physician." *JAMA.* 254(20):2926–2929, 1985.

94. Bernstein, 2001.

95. Bernstein, 2001.

96. Bernstein, 2001.

97. Jonsen, Albert. *The Birth of Bioethics.* New York: Oxford University Press, 1998.

98. Burack, Jeffrey H.; Irby, David; Carline, Jan D.; Root, Richard K.; Larson, Eric B. "Teaching compassion and respect: Attending physicians' responses to problematic behaviors." *Journal of General Internal Medicine.* 14(1):49–55, 1999.

99. Branch, William T. "Supporting the moral development of medical students." *Journal of General Internal Medicine.* 15(7):503–508, 2000.

100. Burack et al., 1999.

101. Burack et al., 1999.

102. Burack et al., 1999.

103. Halpern, Jodi. *From Detached Concern to Empathy: Humanizing Medical Practice.* Oxford, UK: Oxford University Press, 2001.

104. Halpern, 2001.

105. Halpern, 2001.

106. Charon, Rita. "Narrative medicine: A model for empathy, reflection, profession, and trust." *JAMA.* 286(15):1897–1902, 2001.

107. Buckman, Robert, and Kason, Yvonne. *How to Break Bad News.* Baltimore, MD: The Johns Hopkins University Press, 1992.

108. Chambers, Tod. *The Fiction of Bioethics.* New York: Routledge, 1999.

109. Kleinman, Arthur; Eisenberg, Leon; and Good, Byron. "Culture, illness, and care: Clinical lessons from anthropologic and cross-cultural research." *Annals of Internal Medicine.* 88(2):251–258, 1978.

110. Charon, 2001.

111. Branch, 2000.

112. Charon, 2001.

113. Wear, Delese. "On white coats and professional development: The formal and the hidden curricula." *Annals of Internal Medicine.* 129(9):734–737, 1998.

114. Wear, 1998.

115. Branch, William T.; Kern, David; Haidet, Paul; Weissmann, Peter; Gracey, Catherine F.; Mitchell, Gary; Inui, Thomas. "Teaching the human dimensions of care in clinical settings." *JAMA.* 286(9):1067–1074, 2001.

116. Hojat, Mohammedreza; Nasca, Thomas J.; Magee, Mike; Feeney Kendra; Pascual, Rudolfo; Urbano, Frank; Gonnella, Joseph S. "A comparison of the personality profiles of internal medicine residents, physician role models, and the general population." *Academic Medicine.* 74(12):1327–1333, 1999.

117. Hojat et al., 1999.

118. Branch et al., 2001.

119. Branch et al., 2001.

120. Branch et al., 2001.

121. Buckman and Kason, 1992.

122. Buckman and Kason, 1992.

123. Reik, Theodor. *Listening with the Third Ear.* New York: Grove Press, Inc., 1948.

124. Gabbard, Glen O., and Menninger, Roy W. "The psychology of the physician." In *Medical Marriages*, eds. Glen O. Gabbard and Roy W. Menninger, Washington, DC: American Psychiatric Press, 1988, pp. 23–38.

125. Katz, Pearl. *The Scalpel's Edge*. Boston: Allyn and Bacon, 1999.

126. Reik, 1948; Lown, Bernard. *The Lost Art of Healing*. New York: Ballantine Books, 1999.

127. Epstein, Mark. *thoughts without a thinker*. New York: Basic Books, 1995.

128. Hallie, Philip. "Satan, evil and good in history". In *Reason and Violence: Philosophical Investigations*, ed. Sherman Stanage, Totowa, NJ: Littlefield, Adams, and Company, 1974, pp. 53–69.

129. Epstein, 1995.

130. Lown, 1999.

131. Epstein, 1995.

132. Novack, Dennis H.; Suchman, Anthony L.; Clark, William; Epstein, Ronald M.; Najberg, Eva; Kaplan, Craig. "Calibrating the physician: Personal awareness and effective patient care." *JAMA*. 278(6):502–509, 1997.

133. Lipson, Michael and Lipson, Abigail. "Psychotherapy and the ethics of attention." *Hastings Center Report*. 26(1):17–22, 1996.

134. Epstein, Ronald. "Mindful practice." *JAMA*. 282(9):833–839, 1999.

135. Masterson, James F. *The Search for the Real Self*. New York: The Free Press, 1988.

136. Masterson, 1988.

137. Novack et al., 1997.

138. Epstein, 1995.

139. Dornfest, Frank. *Balint Training: A how-to manual in development*. The American Balint Society, undated.

140. Dornfest, undated.

141. Scheingold, Lee. Introduction to Balint seminars. The American Balint Society, undated.

142. Dornfest, undated.

143. Dornfest, undated.

144. Dornfest, undated.

145. Benner, Patricia; Tanner, Christine; Chesla, Catherine. *Expertise in Nursing Practice: Caring, Clinical Judgment, and Ethics*. New York: Springer, 1996.

146. Branch et al., 2001.

147. Novack et al., 1997.

148. Millon, Theodore. *Disorder of Personality: DSM-IV and Beyond*. New York: John Wiley & Sons, Inc., 1996, pp. 393–427.

149. Millon, 1996.

150. Novack, 1997.

151. Novack, 1997.

152. Smith, Martin L., and Forster, Heidi P. "Morally managing medical mistakes." *Cambridge Quarterly of Healthcare Ethics.* 9(1):38–53, 2000.

153. Tsang, Jo-Ann. "Moral rationalization and the integration of situational factors and psychological processes in immoral behavior." *Review of General Psychology.* 6(1):25–50, 2002.

154. Tsang, 2002.

155. Tsang, 2002.

156. Sharpe, Virginia A. "Science, bioethics, and the public interest: On the need for transparency." *Hastings Center Report.* 32(3):23–26, 2002.

Chapter 7

The Empathic Disclosure of Medical Error

John Banja
Geri Amori

"The task of breaking bad news is a testing ground for the entire range of our professional skills and abilities. If we do it badly, the patients or family members may never forgive us; if we do it well, they will never forget us."[1, p. 209]

Robert Buckman and Yvonne Kason

Introduction

The disclosure of harm-causing medical error can be one of the most anguishing experiences a health professional encounters in his or her career.[2] Indeed, it is precisely because error disclosure can be so emotionally painful—punctuated by the professional's experience of intense feelings of having betrayed the patient, the humiliation of having committed or been involved with the error, and fear that the error disclosure will result in some form of penalty—that health providers need to combine effective communication skills with a sound disclosure strategy so that an already unfortunate situation does not become worse.

The material presented here assumes a situation in which individuals with organizational authority agree that a harm-causing error indeed occurred and intend to disclose the error to the harmed individual(s) in a truthful and reasonably comprehensive manner. Given those assumptions, this chapter will discuss important considerations in developing communication strategies and techniques that might prove helpful for disclosing a harm-causing medical error. The strategies discussed result from a synthesis of three sources of reflection and research: the rather large body of literature on conducting empathic communications; the lesser but still considerable amount of literature on how to conduct emotionally painful communications; and the rather scant literature on error disclosure policies. The first part of this chapter will examine some generic considerations about "empathic" communications, why an empathic approach is desirable, and how an empathic approach might permeate the error disclosure communication. The second part will discuss the dialogical specifics of the error disclosure itself.

PART I ■ THE EMPATHIC MODEL

In their classic text, *How to Break Bad News*, Robert Buckman and Yvonne Kason note that emotionally painful conversations are inevitable in healthcare, yet they are often done poorly because many health professionals are not trained in how to conduct them.[3] Not surprisingly, conducting emotionally uncomfortable conversations requires considerable but learnable skill to do well. Disclosing harm-causing medical error falls squarely into the bailiwick of emotionally painful conversations, and many of the points that follow are indebted to Buckman and Kason's work on the empathic delivery of bad news.

Perhaps the first point to make about conducting emotionally painful conversations is that they generally exhibit an iterative stimulus-response psychodynamic. That is, the health provider/communicator is confronted with a situation that provokes uncomfortable feelings and must then manage those feelings simultaneously with his or her conversation. This "feeling-uncomfortable-while-managing-the-communication" phenomenon often pervades the entire communication. *The communication challenge in any bad news conversation is to prevent negative, uncomfortable feelings from compromising the health provider's ability to manage the conversation in a supportive and compassionate way.*[4]

When an emotionally painful conversation centers on the disclosure of a serious medical error, this can be extremely difficult. The aforementioned feelings of fear, anxiety, embarrassment, and so forth can cause the health professional to omit crucial information, to sugar-coat or disrespect the gravity of the situation, to dismiss or ignore the harmed party's questions or feelings, or to manage the conversation in a clumsy, insensitive way (e.g., by dominating the conversation, incessantly interrupting the patient, lecturing, or being defensive).[5]

A fact that often goes unappreciated in conducting painful conversations is how the healthcare professional brings the entirety of his or her psychological formation to every patient or client encounter, and how the attitudes and sensibilities that constitute that formation can be profoundly assaulted in an error disclosure conversation. For example, health providers who take great pride in their attentiveness to detail and competitive success can be humiliated by the commission of a serious medical error. Or the health professional who is easily upset by a patient's emotionality and so prefers to steer clear of emotional content can have an extremely difficult time disclosing error in a truthful and comprehensive fashion. The health professional who needs to be needed or admired among his or her peers and patients can seriously falter in a conversation wherein that need can be profoundly disappointed. And, of course, the health professional who lives in fear of being sued might have to summon enormous moral courage to disclose harm-causing error in a truthful, comprehensive, and prompt fashion.[6]

The fact that these needs and interests can be so compromised in an error disclosure conversation explains why an empathic model is so useful and desirable. That is, the degree of emotional discomfort that professionals feel might unwittingly and unintentionally cause them to focus their attention primarily *on themselves* rather than on the feelings of the listener(s). As Clark and LaBeff note in their paper on delivering news of a patient's death, "You have to be aware of your own feelings and biases because if you don't [sic], you'll wind up dealing with yourself first and the other people second. This isn't the best way to do it."[7, p. 17] But persons who have been harmed from serious medical error naturally want their needs and interests dealt with first.[8] As Buckman and Kason note, persons who are exposed to dreadful news want to feel acknowledged, heard, and validated. Above all, they want their feelings to be deeply respected.[9]

The utility of the empathic approach consists in how it assists professionals to manage their feelings in a way that maintains their concentration on and respect for the feelings *of the harmed party*. A deep appreciation of how the listener is *affectively processing* the conversation is a hallmark of empathic communication.[10] The empathic communicator will be keenly attentive to, guided by, and respectful of the listener's "psychic reality"—that is, how the listener is creating, taking, and sensing the meaning of what he or she is hearing. The empathic communicator will know what to say and how to deliver the message in a way that unwaveringly respects the gravity of the situation and the listener's reactions. (See the various characterizations of empathy in Exhibit 7–1.) An empathic approach maintains the "patient-centeredness" of the conversation and is of enormous value in attenuating the emotional trauma that can result from any bad news communication.[11]

Exhibit 7–1 *Characterizations of Empathy**

"[A] two-way street in which the distinct affective associations of individuals interact and mutually shape each other to yield new thought." (p. 41)

"[An] experiential understanding of another person's distinct emotional perspective." (p. 68)

"[Imagining/understanding] what is salient from (another's) interior perspective." (p. 69)

"[A] first-person experiential knowledge of an agent anticipating her own acts." (p. 73)

"An essentially experiential understanding of another person that involves an active, yet not necessarily voluntary, creation of an interpretive context." (p. 77)

"[I]magining how it feels to experience something." (p. 85)

*Taken from Jodi Halpern's book, From Detached Concern to Empathy (Oxford, UK: Oxford University Press, 2001)

Psychiatrist and ethicist Jodi Halpern remarked, "The empathizer must be in a mood that is interested in the human predicament that another faces."[12, p. 76] Unfortunately, that degree of interest, mood, and attunement to the feelings of the harmed party is rather different from what the literature reports is often found among the communicational styles of nonpsychiatric health professionals. For example, certain physicians and especially surgeons are often known not to engage in conversation at all but rather to dominate their talk with patients and only engage patients with rather close-ended, frequently "yes-no" questions.[13] However, if the essence of a conversation is, as Buckman and Kason suggest, to be guided by the talk itself rather than some preset, professional agenda, then conversations wherein the professional mainly asks close-ended questions, informs the patient of what is going to occur, offers the patient a one-time opportunity to ask questions, and then answers those questions in a curt fashion that discourages further discussion are not conversations at all. Those types of communication will be troublesome in highly emotionally charged situations, yet nonempathic communicators can easily and unthinkingly resort to whatever communicational style feels most comfortable to them and to which they are accustomed. (For a brief list of empathic and nonempathic responses, see Exhibit 7–2.)

Studies of physician-patient communications indicate that patients generally want more discussion about the "meaning" of their illness and how it affects their lives, in contrast to the physician's interest in identifying and treating the disease process.[14] But if health professionals want to establish therapeutic relationships with their patients, they must attend carefully not only to what the patient says but to the emotional tenor or "affect" of the patient's talk. Admittedly, saying, "This must be dreadful for you to hear," to the patient who is obviously distressed upon hearing bad news might subject the communicator to additional emotionality from the patient, which can be very unpleasant for the professional. Indeed, this projection of the patient's emotional pain or anguish onto the health professional is probably the principal reason why many health professionals resist exploring their patients' expressions of psychological or emotional distress.[15] The empathically skillful communicator, however, will be able to, "tolerate emotions that transiently threaten self-esteem … [and] has been educated to cultivate emotional attentiveness to others as part of her own long-term success."[16, p. 61]

The individual who discloses medical error, then, must be psychologically prepared to absorb the listener's shock, anguish, astonishment, bewilderment, or rage and not react defensively. Furthermore, he or she must bear in mind the following, extraordinarily important maxim: "The health professional can safely assume nothing as to how the news will be received."[17, p. 17] Although this may sound like a straightforward contradiction of what has just been said about the need to appreciate how the patient is affectively absorbing the information, it is not, for two reasons. The first is that by imagining how the patient *will* receive the news, the professional substitutes his or her own psychological history for the patient's. But the focus of empathic communication subordinates the communicator's psyche to the listener's. A person's reaction to possibly catastrophic news is learned and derives from the way his or her response was shaped

Exhibit 7-2 *Empathic Techniques and Responses*

Acknowledge:	"This must be .... (dreadful, awful, depressing, frightening) .... for you to hear."
	"This is obviously making you feel very ....."
	"I hear you."
	"That's a very important question."
Listen:	Nonverbal acknowledgment; body language expressing attention to what the other is saying; good eye contact; refraining from interrupting.
Probe:	"Tell me more about that."
	"And how did you experience (or feel about) that? What was that like?"
	"So, this must have caused/must be causing you a lot of .... (heartache, sadness)."
	"I wonder what you're feeling right now."
	"What is it about that that ... (worries, upsets) .... you?"
	"What is it about talking about that ... (you don't like? Makes you anxious? Makes you want to talk about something else?"))
	"What would you like to have happen from this?"
	"How would you like for me to proceed with this information? Are you the sort of person who likes to know the details, or just the big picture? And is there anyone else you'd like me to discuss this with?"
	"Anything else?"
Clarify/Reiterate:	"Now let me make sure I'm understanding you. You're asking me ... (whether or not, how it is that) ..... Is that correct?"
	"So, what you're saying is that ..."
	Repeat the other's last three or four words.

Nonempathic responses

"I know how you feel."

"Try to cheer up. These things happen."

"Maybe this is a blessing in disguise."

"Try to pull yourself together."

"It looks like you'll just have to tough it out."

"I'm sorry you feel that way."

"Perhaps this is God's will."

"Anybody could have screwed this up."

"It wasn't entirely our fault. If your loved had taken better care of himself ... "

Long-winded advising, sermonizing, or lecturing

by nature and nurture.[18] The listener might respond to learning about a harm-causing error with varying degrees of bitterness, shame, despondency, alarm, anxiety, panic, timidity, helplessness, paralysis, confusion, disgust, or shock. But unless the professional has actually seen the listener respond to emotionally difficult situations in the past, he or she will have little idea as to how the individual will respond to the error disclosure. Consequently, communicators must try very hard to concentrate on and assess how the listener is reacting to the disclosure, rather than ask themselves, "How would *I* react to this news?" By respecting, acknowledging, and going with the listener's reaction, the communicator will be better able to resist excusing, defending, or rationalizing the error, and the temptation to de-emphasize or, much worse, dismiss the significance or appropriateness of the listener's response.[19]

The second reason why communicators should not assume how the news is going to be received is that doing so can easily upset their articulation or delivery. The communicator who is worried about how the listener will respond 5 or 10 or 15 seconds into the error disclosure may falter, stutter, hedge, or obfuscate the communication according to the stress he or she is experiencing.[20] The best technique for initiating a bad news conversation is for the communicator to:

1) Rehearse his or her disclosure of the information
2) Deliver it as simply, truthfully, and economically as possible
3) Stop talking
4) Assess how the news is being received
5) Respond empathically[21]

Many communicators, especially if they are physicians, experience two profound temptations that must be resisted during the disclosure of medical error. The first is for the health professional to simply keep talking. As noted, nonpsychiatric physicians often dominate their discussions with patients.[22] Indeed, any authority figure who is used to being deferred to as an expert, who is accustomed to interrupting but not being interrupted, and who uses language as a medium or token of his or her authority might be sorely tempted to continue talking throughout an emotionally challenging communication and not allow the listener to get a word in edgewise. This temptation will be especially strong during moments of silence, which often make physicians uncomfortable.

Empathic communicators, on the other hand, pay special attention to "silent" communication. In error disclosure scenarios, the communicator's respect for silence by refraining from interjecting random conversation simply to relieve emotional discomfort shows concern for the listener and the importance of the situation. Silence respects the gravity of the situation whereas talking for the sake of lightening the participants' mood can easily backfire, as when, for example, someone makes a humorous remark that no one else finds amusing.[23, pp.158-159] Throughout the conversation, error disclosers should take their conversational cues from their listeners and allow the conversation to go where *the listener* wishes to take it.[24] After all, the error disclosure communication is for the sake of the listener, not the health professional.

Despite the necessity to conduct such conversations artfully and skillfully, it is lamentable that nonpsychiatric health professionals often have no specific training in empathic communications and thus find themselves at the mercy of their (possibly undisciplined) emotional reactions to stressful situations.[25] For many health providers, empathic communication is an utterly foreign way of talking.[26] But if there is any lesson to be gained from various studies on malpractice litigation, it is that many lawsuits are precipitated by poor or absent communications.[27] A frequently cited study by Gerald Hickson and his colleagues at Vanderbilt revealed, for example, that 20 percent of the litigants surveyed claimed they were suing largely to find out what happened—so brusque, distant, and uncommunicative had their health providers become when an untoward outcome occurred.[28] Alternatively, if the communicator can fashion his or her error disclosure conversation in a way so that listeners feel heard, acknowledged, and respected throughout, the communication will have been successful regardless of whether it proceeds to litigation or not. After all, communicators can control only how they represent the error scenario to the harmed parties and the extent to which they maintain support for their listeners. What the harmed parties do after the communication is beyond the control of the health professional.

The following provides concrete suggestions as to how the disclosure of harm-causing error might proceed.

PART II ■ HOW TO DISCLOSE

Initial Considerations

1. *Agree on what happened.* Before error disclosure can occur, the communicators must not only agree that harm-causing error took place, but they must also agree on all of the pertinent facts involving the error's commission and aftermath. This not only means that whoever ultimately discloses the error to the harmed party should possess exquisite familiarity with what happened, but that the error discloser's version of "what happened" is shared by all the other professionals in the room.[29, p. 50] Obviously, risk management plays a crucial role in constructing the "reality" or circumstances of the error and can help the communicators to agree on the essential moments of the error trajectory. A common recommendation, therefore, is that *before error is disclosed to the harmed party, the health professionals should report the error to risk management, which in turn should launch an investigation into what occurred.* If that investigation quickly confirms the fact that harm-causing error occurred, then the error should be disclosed to the harmed party. If it is uncertain that an error occurred or that the error caused the patient's harm, the health professional should counter any anxious questions from the patient or the family by saying something like, "Mr. Jones, what happened was so

terribly unexpected and to make matters worse, we are uncertain as to what caused this. But please know we are investigating this right now and as soon as we know what happened, we will certainly tell you."

2. *Who should be present?* It remains a matter of speculation and debate as to which professionals should make up the error disclosure team as well as who can best serve the role of principal communicator. Whereas some organizations prefer an administrator to do the disclosure, most of the literature suggests that the harmed party's attending physician be the principal communicator.[30, pp. 38, 43, 49] If the attending, however, is known to be a generally poor speaker, or lacks good communication skills in the listener's primary language, or is emotionally distraught, then he or she is a poor candidate. A suggestion worth considering is to have the health professional with whom the harmed party had the best relationship serve either as the principal or secondary communicator.[31, p. 49] Of course, if the harmed party is unable to be present or is cognitively or psychologically incapacitated so that he or she cannot meaningfully participate in the conversation, the disclosure should be made to the harmed party's legal proxy or surrogate, who will probably be a spouse or some other immediate next of kin.

Although it is a matter of debate, it might be preferable to excuse the hospital's or institution's legal counsel from the initial conversation. The presence of an attorney might cast an adversarial tone on the proceedings that, at least at the initial error disclosure conversation, ought to be avoided. On the other hand, an institutional representative should be present to ensure that the disclosure is communicated in a truthful and reasonably comprehensive manner.

3. *Where should the disclosure occur?* Although many institutions prefer that the error disclosure conversation occur on institutional premises, serious consideration should be given to holding the conversation at the harmed party's residence or preferred venue. The point, of course, is to make the conversational environment as accommodating as possible to those who are to receive the news.

4. *Tape recorders.* A question sometimes arises as to whether the error disclosure conversation should be audio-taped. We believe the best approach is for the communicators to follow the lead of the listeners. That is, if the listeners produce a tape recorder and insist on audiotaping the conversation, we suggest that the communicators also audiotape the conversation to ensure its reliability. Although some hospitals have a policy that prohibits taping error disclosure conversations, the hospital's administrators should consider how this policy might anger the listeners and rupture the communication from the outset.

5. *The setting.* If the disclosure occurs on institutional premises, it is best for it to take place in a private, quiet room.[32] One of the unfortunate realities of bad news communications, such as the disclosure of a terminal disease or even a death disclosure, is that they sometimes occur in obtrusively public places, for example, waiting rooms, busy hallways, or in front of hospital elevators. If the communication is about harm-causing medical error, the communicators should not be distracted by phones, beepers, fax machines, or ambient noise such as hallway conversations.

The room should not be cramped but should have considerable space in case one of the listeners wants to stand up and walk around—a not unusual reaction to hearing bad news. Buckman and Kason suggest that there not be a desk in the room because certain kinds of furniture influence mood and perceptions of power.[33, p. 46] The healthcare provider who sits on one side of a desk suggests an "us-versus-them" climate, which is obviously inadvisable.

6. Anticipate being sued. A suggestion that error disclosers should well consider when commencing the error disclosure conversation is to fully expect that no matter how skillfully and empathically the communication is delivered, and no matter how well the harmed party displays emotional control, the institution will be sued. Even though lawsuits often do not transpire when the error is disclosed truthfully and empathically, anticipating that a lawsuit will nevertheless occur might calm the communicators in a way that facilitates empathy. And while it is easier said than done, appreciating the fact that error disclosure is the right thing to do regardless of its consequences might lighten some of the burden associated with disclosure.

Talking and Listening

1. Body language. One of the cardinal mistakes that bad news communicators are often accused of is standing throughout the entire conversation while the listeners sit. In empathic conversations the communicators should not only sit, but should also adjust their eye level to be somewhat lower than the listeners.[34, p. 142] The effect this has upon listeners is a communication of respect, as the harmed parties perceive the primary communicator to be looking up to them.

Bad news communicators must also pay attention to their physical posture and vocal delivery of information.[35] The communicator who sits rigidly upright on the edge of the chair with knees tightly closed and hands clasped in his or her lap is unlikely to communicate calm to the listeners. An empathic position is one wherein the communicator sits and leans slightly forward, shoulders slumped or slouched, knees apart, with forearms resting comfortably on the legs.[36, pp. 45–46]

Most listeners desire direct eye contact—because it communicates an "I am acknowledging you" message—although individuals from certain cultures (e.g., Native Americans) may not.[37] Facial expression, especially the eyebrows and line of the lips or set of the jaw, should convey contriteness and gentleness but not intensity, which can be mistaken for anger. Deeply furrowed eyebrows, pursed lips, and speaking through a tightly clenched jaw are not recommended.

2. Talking. When unpracticed individuals are agitated and must speak, they will often talk rapidly or stutter, splutter, or mumble. Their vocal volume might verge toward the inaudible or ear-splitting. They might also be tremendously tempted to interrupt often if they feel defensive or challenged, and once they start talking, they might not be able to stop. The empathic communicator will make brief remarks and frequently stop speaking, as this gives the listeners time to digest what has been said or to ask questions.[38]

3. How to begin. After ensuring that appropriate introductions are made for all present, the communicator should begin with something like:

> Mr. Jones, what I have to tell you is going to be difficult for me to say and probably very hard for you to hear. However, while you/your family member was receiving treatment here, there was a mistake made in the course of your/his/her care. Now, I'm wondering how you'd like me to proceed with this information. Would you like to know what occurred, or is there another way you'd prefer I communicate the information?"

There are a number of features of this opening—which is a variant of one that Buckman and Kason recommend in breaking bad news—that merit attention. The first sentence is what the literature calls a "warning shot." It alerts the listener to the fact that what follows is not going to be good news, and it gives the communicator a brief, albeit perhaps valuable, moment to articulate some words, listen to the sound of his or her voice, and get settled.[39]

The second sentence contains the word "mistake" (or "error"). We believe it is essential for the error discloser to say either of these words. Other terms such as "complication" or "misadventure" are vague, even obfuscatory, and disrespect the listener's right to know what happened.[40] The primary reason for the meeting is to disclose the fact that error has occurred. Hence, the words "mistake" or "error" should be enunciated no matter how painful they are to say. Trying to describe a harm-causing error in a truthful, factual, and objective manner without saying "error" or "mistake" invites the listener to ask, "So, then, you made a mistake? You screwed up! You're telling me you people made a big mistake? Right?" But forcing the listener to draw that inference may make him or her more upset over the communicator's unwillingness to call a spade a spade. Worse, the communicator who looks anxiously at his or her colleagues when asked whether a mistake was made and then replies, "Well, we don't like to use that word," is courting relational disaster.

This means that the traditional advice given by insurance carriers to resist using "liability" sounding words such as "error" or "mistake" is, we suggest, wrong because it denies the harmed party's right to know the truth. Indeed, it is worth wondering whether the reluctance of health providers to explain what happened in a compassionate and reasonably comprehensive manner in any number of adverse outcomes scenarios, whether they are caused by error or not, is a significant, contributing factor to the malpractice crisis physicians are experiencing today.

The third sentence respects the listener's right to control the conversation and determine its direction. There is no telling how the listener will respond. He or she might demand a comprehensive, highly detailed account of what happened, or just want to hear a brief description of the events. He or she might want to terminate the conversation early on, acknowledge the communicators, walk out of the room, and never return.

Or the listener might want to schedule another meeting, perhaps with his or her lawyer present. The point of the "How would you like me to proceed?" question, though, is thoroughly in keeping with an empathic sensibility of respecting the listener's affective understanding of what is going on and honoring his or her preferences over how the conversation should proceed.[41]

4. The telephonic disclosure. In some instances, the first contact with the harmed party or his or her representative will be telephonic. Here, the error communicator may well be inclined to analogize this situation to a telephonic death disclosure wherein only enough information is conveyed to encourage the listener to come to the hospital but without disclosing the entire truth about what happened. Just as some of the anecdotal evidence on telephonic communications of an unanticipated death indicates that listeners are encouraged to come to the facility as soon as possible but are not told about the patient's death until they arrive, so the telephonic error discloser might similarly hesitate to communicate any information beyond his or her interest in scheduling a meeting.[42]

Error disclosers should be aware of a serious pitfall in this approach, which is that the listener might press the caller for reasons for the meeting. If the caller says, "Mrs. Jones, this is Dr. Smith from Ajax Hospital where your father received care some days ago. I was wondering if you might drop by my office tomorrow around 3:00. There are some things I'd like to discuss with you," the caller risks Mrs. Jones asking, "What kind of things? What are you talking about?" And even if Mrs. Jones initially accepts the 3:00 invitation with no questions asked, Dr. Smith's phone might ring five minutes later with Mrs. Jones on the other end asking questions. If Dr. Smith hesitates and says, "Well, Mrs. Jones, I'd really prefer not to discuss that right now," he risks provoking or angering Mrs. Jones.

We encourage the caller to be *prepared* to tell virtually everything, but to give the listener a chance to control the amount of telephonic conversational material.[43] Thus, the telephonic conversation might begin like this:

> Mrs. Jones, the reason I'm calling is to discuss with you, or with whomever you'd like, something we've learned about your father's care while he was here. Would you like me to go into the details right now, or would you prefer to wait until we can set up a face-to-face meeting?

This is a much more empathic approach as it allows Mrs. Jones to control the conversation. Remember, the communicator must resist anticipating how the listener will respond and should instead trust the listener to decide what is in his or her best interests to hear, and how much information he or she can tolerate. Also and very importantly, the literature has long reported that health providers tend to underestimate the amount of psychological discomfort upon hearing bad news that patients or family members can tolerate.[44] In fact, the contemporary interpretation of the health provider who says, "Oh, we can't tell the patient what happened; he would be psychologically unable to tolerate the news," is that the health provider is the one with a psychological intolerance problem, and is transferring that discomfort onto the patient.[45]

5. *The content of the disclosure*. Borrowing from a number of sources, it is suggested that the content of the disclosure include the items listed in Exhibit 7–3. Throughout the conversation, though, it is crucial for the communicator to:

- Answer questions truthfully and honestly; do not hedge or rationalize and, above all, do not talk "medicalese"[46]
- Apologize for what happened [47, pp. 46, 51, and 63]
- Maintain eye contact except if the listener cries, then do not stare; also, have a box of Kleenex handy[48]
- Stop frequently, as this gives the listener permission to ask questions[49]
- Refrain from sugar-coating the news or dismissing the gravity of what happened[50, pp. 38 and 43]
- Be led by the listener's cues, questions, and feelings and direct the conversation according to the listener's agenda[51]
- Resist the urge to interrupt, especially if the listener becomes irate or accusatory; in these instances, it is best for the communicator to maintain silence and/or contriteness[52, p. 50]
- Anticipate numerous moments of feeling vulnerable and wretched[53]

6. *Managing emotional outbursts or other unsavory moments*. At no time should the communicator admonish the listener's behavior unless that behavior appears harm-

Exhibit 7–3 *Content of the Error Disclosure*

- A description of the nature of the error and the harm it caused
- When and where the error occurred
- Consequence of the harm
- Clinical and institutional actions taken to diminish the gravity of the harm
- Actions taken to prevent future occurrences of the error
- Who will manage the patient's continuing care
- Identification of systemic elements that contributed to the error
- Who will manage ongoing communications
- Associated costs of the error to be removed from the patient's bill (assuming these costs are known to be related to the error and risk management has been consulted)
- Offer of counseling and support

ful to the listener (such as overt suicidality) or to the communicator (such as overt homicidality).

It is understandable for communicators to dread listeners' reactions such as, "You're telling me you killed my father?!" The best response to this question might very well be, "I'm sorry beyond words to say that that is probably what happened." Or the listener might scream, "Let me tell you something, you bastards. By the time this is over, I'm going to own this hospital!" The best response to this might very well be a quiet, "I'm so terribly sorry, Mr./Ms. ...."

It is suggested that the nearest communicators come to making a defensive remark is saying something like, "Mr. X, we felt we had to tell you the truth about this error. We believe it would have been wrong to conceal this information from you. Of course, that doesn't make it any easier for you to hear. Again, we are so deeply sorry this has happened." Notice how this response keeps the emotional spotlight on the listeners, which is what an empathic communication should do, in contrast to a statement like, "Mr. X, don't you realize how difficult it is for us to tell you this? Not only is it horrible for us, but we're taking a risk that you might sue us." This latter response turns the spotlight on the communicators' feelings, which might not only be of little importance to the listener, but might strike him or her as dismissing the pain he or she is experiencing.

7. Refrain from blame. A fine but firm line ought to be drawn between telling what happened in a truthful and comprehensive fashion versus identifying "blameworthy" parties with a detailed description of their mistakes.[54, p. 52] Thus, in disclosing a serious medication error to Ms. Jones, the communicator might tell her that a prescription was written for the patient to have 10 milligrams of X but she was actually given 100 milligrams, which probably caused her to experience Y. If Mrs. Jones asks how that happened, she should be told that the prescription was misread and that the usual system checks or fail-safe mechanisms did not detect the error. The communicators should refrain from blaming specific error operators, such as saying, "Dr. Williams's handwriting on the prescription was illegible, so Nurse Conrad got together with some other nurses on the floor and they took their best guess."

Following the contemporary ideology of the systemic nature of error, we suggest that when the error is clearly a systemic one, blame for the error should be collectivized or shared, meaning that it be assumed by the institution.[55] A good response to a harmed party's probing for names and specific details (and that might have to be repeated during the course of the conversation) is, "Ms. Jones, we very much want you to know that the harm your father experienced was no one, single person's fault. The system failed, and we deeply regret it."

8. Apologize profusely. Anecdotal evidence indicates that many health providers resist apologies because they fear it is tantamount to an admission of negligence. As noted in previous chapters, however, harmed parties very much want to hear an apology.[56] Heartfelt apologizing tends to defuse anger, and it tokens categorical respect. A frequently cited study found that 37 percent of patients suing health providers claimed they would not have instigated a malpractice action had they received an explanation of what happened and an apology.[57] Furthermore, if the communicator tells the listener what occurred and admits error, omitting an apology seems remarkably insensitive.

9. "*Associated costs of the error will be removed from the bill.*" We believe it is crucial to include this in the error disclosure.[58, p.55] Externalizing whatever costs occur from the error to the harmed party is emphatically not one of the contractual obligations a patient assumes in the professional-patient relationship. As with any other professional relationship wherein the consumer has experienced injury or financial loss from treatment that fell below the professional standard, the professional has an obligation to "make it right." Mentioning the omission of costs connected with the error from the patient's bill is not only respectful, but it might mollify feelings of vindictiveness or rage that some listeners will have.

10. *Planning and follow-through*. A key consideration of an error disclosure meeting is the distinct possibility that it will not be the last such encounter with the harmed party. Consequently, communicators should provide contact information for institutional personnel whom the harmed parties can call upon for further discussion.[59, pp. 51 and 64]

The possibility that the harmed party might desire additional meetings or that, at least, he or she will replay the meeting numerous times in his or her experiential memory should reinforce the communicators' intentions to act as empathically and respectfully as possible. Regardless of whether the listener reacts with civility or fury during the meeting, he or she may be profoundly and positively influenced by how respected he or she was by the staff throughout the conversation, especially if there were moments when he or she lost emotional control.

Ultimately, the pragmatic value of empathy consists in preventing a relationship that has been marred by a misfortune like harm-causing error from worsening. This doubtlessly explains why a compassionate and respectful disclosure of error often does not result in a malpractice action or that when it does, cases are known to settle speedily and at a fraction of the amount that juries have been known to award to plaintiffs— especially to ones who were able to show that their medical misfortunes were dismissed or ignored by seemingly "uncaring" health providers.[60]

11. *Empathy for the error operators*. Although providing support to the error operators is not exactly a dimension of the error disclosure conversation itself, we would be remiss not to mention it. The admission, reporting, and disclosure of a serious medical error can be utterly traumatic to the involved professionals. Institutions should offer them profound support, not unlike what is offered to any employee in need of help with a trying life challenge.[61]

Conclusion

As noted previously, Section 8.12 of *The Current Opinions of the AMA Code of Ethics* aptly articulates the moral reasons for error disclosure:

It is a fundamental ethical requirement that a physician should at all times deal honestly and openly with patients. Patients have a right to know their past and present medical status and to be free of any mistaken beliefs concerning their conditions. Situations occasionally occur in which a patient suffers significant medical complications that may have resulted from the physician's mistake or judgment. In these situations, the physician is ethically required to inform the patient of all the facts necessary to ensure understanding of what has occurred. Only through full disclosure is a patient able to make informed decisions regarding future medical care.[62, pp. 217-218]

Whereas many if not most health professionals would concur with these sensibilities, relatively few of them have been systematically taught the empathic, communicational strategies and insights outlined in this chapter. Even so, it is hardly enough to read and think about the strategies described here. They must be practiced. Health professionals who are intent on improving their empathic skills must constantly monitor their performance and ask themselves what they could have done better. These professionals would do well to seek feedback from others who might have been present at such conversations. Indeed, videotaping and then critiquing practice sessions on the delivery of bad news can take a professional's empathic skills to a new level of expertise.

Ultimately, the ability of health professionals to communicate empathically when disclosing harm-causing error will derive from their ego strength—that is, their psychical ability to withstand the censuring of their consciences, the emotional assault they might have to endure from an individual who is shocked about the commission of the error and its subsequent harm, and the fear they can feel in contemplating the aftermath of the error disclosure.[63, pp. 192-197] Securing and maintaining that ego strength, however, requires a deep institutional commitment to those professionals charged with error disclosure. Judith Andre notes that ethics is largely about doing the right thing, for the right reasons, supported by the right feelings.[64] We suggest that the empathic approach resonates with and perhaps even grounds these components of right action, especially as it extends not only to the harmed parties but to those professionals disclosing the error. When a harm-causing error rears its head, institutions that practice empathy with their patients as well as their staff will be best poised to meet the psychological and communicational challenges that "doing the right thing" presents.

References

1. Buckman, Robert, and Kason, Yvonne. *How to Break Bad News*. Baltimore, MD: Johns Hopkins University Press, 1992.
2. Christensen, John F.; Levinson, Wendy; Dunn, Patrick M. "The heart of darkness: The impact of perceived mistakes on physicians." *Journal of General Internal Medicine*. 7(July/August):424–431, 1992; Wu, Albert W.; Folkman, Susan; McPhee, Stephen J; Lo, Bernard. "How house officers cope with their

mistakes." *Western Journal of Medicine.* 159(5):565–569, 1993; Wolf, Zane Robinson. *Medication Errors: The Nursing Experience.* Albany, NY: Delmar Publishers, Inc., 1994; Smith, Martin L. and Forster, Heidi P. "Morally managing medical mistakes." *Cambridge Quarterly of Healthcare Ethics.* 9(1): 38–53, 2000; Thurman, Andrew E. "Institutional responses to medical mistakes: ethical and legal perspectives." *Kennedy Institute of Ethics Journal.* 11(2):147–156, 2001; Nowicki, Michael and Chaku, Maneesh. "Do healthcare managers have an ethical duty to admit mistakes?" *Healthcare Financial Management.* October:64–66, 1998.

3. Buckman and Kason, 1992.

4. Ptacek, J. T., and Eberhardt, Tara L. "Breaking bad news: A review of the literature." *JAMA.* 276(6):496–502, 1996.

5. Buckman and Kason, 1992; Finkelstein, Daniel; Wu, Albert W; Holtzman, Neil A.; Smith, Melanie K. "When a physician harms a patient by a medical error: Ethical, legal and risk-management considerations." *The Journal of Clinical Ethics.* 8(4):330–335, 1997.

6. Katz, Pearl. *The Scalpel's Edge.* Needham Heights, MA: Allyn & Bacon, 1999; Hilfiker, David. "Sounding board: Facing our mistakes." *New England Journal of Medicine.* 310(2):118–324, 1984; Lazarus, Richard S., and Folkman, Susan. *Stress, Appraisal, and Coping.* New York: Springer Verlag, Inc., 1984; University HealthSystem Consortium. *Shining the Light on Errors: How Open Should We Be?* Oak Brook, IL: University Health System Consortium, 2002.

7. Clark, R. E., and LaBeff, E. E. "Death telling: Managing the delivery of bad news." Quoted in Iserson, Kenneth V. *Grave Words.* Tucson, AZ: Galen Press, Ltd., 1998.

8. Vincent, Charles; Young, Magi; Phillips, Angela. "Why do people sue doctors? A study of patients and relatives taking legal action." *Lancet.* 343(8913): 609–613, 1994; Hingorani, Melanie; Wong, Tina; and Vafidis, Gilli. "Patients' and doctors' attitudes to amount of information given after unintended injury during treatment." *British Medical Journal.* 318(7184):640–641, 1999; Buller, M. K., Buller, D. B. "Physicians' communication style and patient satisfaction." *Journal of Health and Social Behavior.* 28:375–388, 1987; Hinds, Cora; Streater, Alicia; Mood, Darlene. "Functions and preferred methods of receiving information related to radiotherapy." *Cancer Nursing.* 18(5):374–384, 1995.

9. Buckman and Kason, 1992.

10. Halpern, Jodi. *From Detached Concern to Empathy.* Oxford: Oxford University Press, 2001.

11. Girgis, Alaf, and Sanson-Fisher, Rob W. "Breaking bad news: Consensus guidelines for medical practitioners." *Journal of Clinical Oncology.* 13(9): 2449–2456, 1995; Davis, Hilton. "Breaking bad news." *Practitioner.* 235 (1503):522–526, 1991; Quill, Timothy, and Townsend, Penelope. "Bad news:

Delivery, dialogue, and dilemmas." *Archives of Internal Medicine.* 151(3): 463–468, 1991; Fallowfield, Lesley J. "Giving sad and bad news." *Lancet.* 341 (8843):476–478, 1993; Miranda, Jeanne, and Brody, Robert. "Communicating bad news." *Western Journal of Medicine.* 156(1):83–85, 1992; Maguire, Peter, and Faulkner, Ann. "Communicating with cancer patients: Handling bad news and difficult questions." *British Medical Journal.* 297(Oct. 8):907–909, 1988.

12. Halpern, 2001.

13. Levinson, Wendy, and Chaumeton, Nigel. "Communication between surgeons and patients in routine office visits." *Surgery.* 125(2):127–134, 1999.

14. Halpern, 2001; Bertakis, Klea; Roter, Debra; and Putnam, Samuel. "The relationship of physician interview style to patient satisfaction." *The Journal of Family Practice.* 32(2):175–181, 1991.

15. Gunther, Meyer. "Catastrophic illness and the caregivers: Real burdens and solutions with respect to the role of the behavioral sciences." In *Rehabilitation Psychology Desk Reference*, ed. Caplan, Bruce. Rockville, MD: Aspen, 1987, pp. 219–243.

16. Halpern, 2001.

17. Buckman and Kason, 1992.

18. Lazarus and Folkman, 1984.

19. Ptacek and Eberhardt, 1996; Colon, K. "Breaking the bad news." *Minnesota Medicine.* 78:10–14, 1995.

20. Lazarus and Folkman, 1984.

21. Nowicki and Chaku, 1993; Buckman and Kason, 1992; Girgis and Sanson-Fisher, 1995; Fallowfield, 1993; Maguire and Faulkner, 1988.

22. Katz, 1999; Levinson and Chaumeton, 1999.

23. Buckman and Kason, 1992.

24. Girgis and Sanson-Fisher, 1995; Davis, 1991; Quill and Townsend, 1991.

25. Buckman and Kason, 1992.

26. Katz, 1999.

27. Hickson, Gerald B.; Clayton, Ellen Wright; Githens, Penny B.; Sloan, Frank A. "Factors that prompted families to file medical malpractice claims following perinatal injuries." *JAMA.* 267(10):1359–1363, 1992.

28. Hickson et al., 1992.

29. University HealthSystem Consortium, 2002.

30. University HealthSystem Consortium, 2002.

31. University HealthSystem Consortium, 2002.

32. Girgis and Sanson-Fisher, 1995; Davis, 1991; Quill and Townsend, 1991.

33. Buckman and Kason, 1992.

34. Buckman and Kason, 1992.

35. Davis, 1991; Quill and Townsend, 1991; Fallowfield, 1993; Davis, H. *Counseling Parents of Children with Chronic Illness or Disability*. London: British Psychological Society, 1993; Brewin, Thurstan. "Three ways of giving bad news." *Lancet*. 337(8751):1207–1209, 1991.

36. Buckman and Kason, 1992.

37. Davis, 1993; Brewin, 1991; Campbell, 1994; Creagan, Edward T. "How to break bad news—and not devastate the patient." *Mayo Clinic Proceedings*. 69(10):1015–1017, 1994.

38. Buckman and Kason, 1992; Hogshead, H. P. "The art of delivering bad news." *Journal of the Florida Medical Association*. 63:807, 1976; Michaels, Evelyne. "Deliver bad news tactfully." *Canadian Medical Association Journal*. 129 (Dec. 15):1307–1308, 1983.

39. Miranda and Brody, 1992; Maguire and Faulkner, 1988; Campbell, 1994; Bor, R.; Miller, R.; Goldman, E.; Scher, I. "The meaning of bad news in HIV disease: Counseling about dreaded issues revisited." *Counseling Psychology Quarterly*. 6:69–80, 1993; Faulkner, A.; Maguire, P.; Regnard, C. "Breaking bad news—a flow diagram." *Palliative Medicine*. 8:145–151, 1994.

40. Hickson et al., 1992.

41. Hogshead, 1976; Michaels, 1983; Falvo, Donna R., and Smith, Jana K. "Assessing residents' behavioral science skills: Patients' views of physician-patient interaction." *Journal of Family Practice*. 17(3):479–483, 1983.

42. Iserson, 1998; Davidhizar, Ruth M., and Monhaut, Nanette. "Giving bad news by phone." *Nursing*. 15(4):58–59, 1985.

43. Falvo and Smith, 1983; Davidhizar and Monhaut, 1985.

44. Hingorani, Wong, and Vafidis, 1999.

45. Katz, 1999.

46. Ptacek and Eberhardt, 1996; Girgis and Sanson-Fisher, 1995.

47. University HealthSystem Consortium, 2002.

48. Buckman and Kason, 1992; Brewin, 1991; Campbell, 1994; Creagan, 1994.

49. Davis, 1991; Quill and Townsend, 1991.

50. University HealthSystem Consortium, 2002; Beasley, N. W.; Wheby, M. S.; Pruett, T. L. "Medical center hour: Breaking the bad news." *Virginia Medical Quarterly*. 120:90–93, 1993.

51. Hogshead, 1976; Michaels, 1983; Falvo and Smith, 1983.

52. Buckman and Kason, 1992.

53. Christensen, Levinson, and Dunn, 1992; Wu, Folkman, McPhee, and Lo, 1993; Wolf, 1994; Smith and Forster, 2000; Thurman, 2001; Nowicki and Chaku, 1998.

54. University HealthSystem Consortium, 2002.

55. Kohn, Linda T.; Corrigan, Janet M.; and Donaldson, Molla S. *To Err Is Human: Building a Safer Health System.* Washington, DC: National Academy Press, 2000.

56. Vincent, Young, and Phillips, 1994; Hingorani, Wong, and Vafidis, 1999.

57. Vincent, Young, and Phillips, 1994.

58. University HealthSystems Consortium, 2002.

59. University HealthSystems Consortium, 2002.

60. Kraman, Steve S., and Hamm, Ginny. "Risk management: Extreme honesty may be the best policy." *Annals of Internal Medicine.* 131(12):963–967, 1999.

61. Wolf, Zane R., and Cohen, Michael. "Caregivers' reactions to making medication errors." In *Medication Errors: Causes, Prevention, and Risk Management,* ed. Cohen, Michael R. Boston, MA: Jones and Bartlett Publishers, 2000, pp. 7.1–7.10.

62. Council on Ethical and Judicial Affairs. *Code of Medical Ethics: Current Opinions with Annotations.* 2002–2003 Edition. Chicago, IL: AMA Press, 2002. AMA, Code of Opinion.

63. Buckman and Kason, 1992.

64. Andre, Judith. "Humility reconsidered." In *Margin of Error: The Ethics of Mistakes in the Practice of Medicine,* eds. Rubin, S. and Zoloth, L. Hagerstown, MD: University Publishing Group, 2000, pp. 59–72.

Chapter 8

Beyond Errors–
Beyond
Narcissism

"Error is the stuff of which the web of life is woven and he who lives longest and wisest is only able to weave out the more of it."[1, p. 219]

Thomas Jefferson

The old pond.

A frog jumps in.

Plop![2, p. 113]

Japanese haiku

I wrote this book with a particular kind of health professional in mind. He or she is one who believes it immensely important to:

- Maintain a professional distance or guardedness with patients that largely precludes empathically reacting to their anxiety or suffering
- Appear utterly competent always
- Understand and ground that competence in scientific method and a densely clinical vocabulary
- Never admit ignorance, hesitation, or error
- Direct and control the conversation with patients always
- Use the power of his or her white coat to direct how the patient should behave and feel

Now, there is abundant anecdotal evidence to suggest that in various degrees and combinations, these characteristics are very common among many health professionals, especially physicians. While this person is hardly the prototypical narcissist that fits the DSM-IV criteria as mentioned in Chapter 3, consider that this individual probably assumes these behaviors because of his staunch belief that they are crucial in keeping both his sense of self and the clinical situations he manages every day from "falling apart." That is, these behaviors and the self-structure that underlie them provide a feeling of cohesion, solidity, and reliability that assuages his fear of losing control or feeling inadequate or helpless. Perhaps just as he believes that his parents wanted him to evince certain behaviors so that he could feel worthwhile and admirable in their eyes, so he similarly believes that his patients want him to appear omniscient, unhesitating, and perhaps even a bit arrogant. There is also an excellent chance that he is an individual who needs to assert his sense of authority; that he believes the professional situation demands deference from his patient-clients; and that, in the name of that professionality, he must maintain a decidedly impersonal relationship with patients that only recognizes their symptoms and those symptoms' causes. He is not known for his warmth, but rather for these very familiar behaviors by which he is indeed admired when things go well, but which often result in his patients' wrath when they go poorly. This person is a medical narcissist, whose hallmark feature is the emotionally distancing behaviors he assumes so as to cope with the stress and anxiety of delivering care. Indeed, the great liability of his character formation is that he might stop differentiating his real self from the professional one he has cultivated. Over time, the medical narcissist might simply come to find the professional self so comforting, pleasing, reliable, effective, and "solid" that, as occurs with all advanced narcissists, he cannot resist merging his real self with this ideal one.

This final chapter addresses how health professionals might be prepared to understand the impact of medical error as a lesson about life and their experience of it. Toward that end, I will liberally use some material from one of my favorite books on narcissism, Mark Epstein's *thoughts without a thinker*. Epstein was a practicing Buddhist before he went to medical school and eventually trained in psychiatry. Because he has practiced Buddhism throughout his adult life, his book contrasts as well as blends certain of Buddhism's most salient lessons with Western approaches to psychotherapy. I also want to buttress Epstein's observations with others from another text I admire, Bernard Lown's *The Lost Art of Healing*, so as to leave the reader with some final impressions about the destructive power of unhealthy narcissism and the life-enrichment possibilities that can result from "overcoming" the self.

The Narcissistically Cohesive Self

Consider the characterization of unhealthy narcissism that was discussed in the third chapter: that a prominent explanation of narcissism posits an idealized self that develops from an individual's identifying only with a preferred or valued set of behaviors, feelings, and beliefs, while other less ideal self-aspects are rejected, denied, suppressed, or projected onto others. This reconstructed narcissistic self feels solid, "together," ample, definitive, and impressive even though this self, like Narcissus's reflection in the pond, is only imagined and not real.

Like all unhealthy narcissists, the medical narcissist who suffers from disrupted self-esteem does not want to experience his real self—that is, the one who admits imperfections, limitations, and anxieties. But because these painful aspects of his real self can never be entirely split off but only repressed or suppressed, the narcissist's denial of them becomes a focal point for the formation of frustration, anger, covetousness, and envy because the narcissist's ideal self is a hopeless fiction. Just as Narcissus's reflection in the pool disappears as he tries to grasp it, so the ideal self is always frustratingly out of reach. Just as unhealthy narcissists idealize those persons whom they want to emulate, they also find themselves competing with those very persons for power and respect. And when those others do not live up to the narcissist's idealized expectations, the narcissist dismisses them, often with a feeling that they have somehow betrayed him.[3]

Epstein points out that people often come into therapy trying to grasp their "true" or "real" self. The more emotionally fragile medical narcissist makes his or her signal mistake in believing that such a self has already been professionally formulated so that all he or she has to do is assimilate it. But that process of assimilation begins with, and indeed is motivated by, a critical miscalculation that recalls one of Freud's central observations about narcissism: that narcissism is a reaction to our inability to tolerate unpleasant truths about ourselves.[4] Indeed, if Gabbard and other psychiatric commentators are right in asserting that the choice of medicine as a profession is an anxiety-generated reaction to the body's ultimate fragility, vulnerability, deterioration, and death, then the unpleasant truth denied by medical narcissists is twofold: not only do they deny their inherent imperfections, but they also ultimately deny their mortality. As Epstein explains:

> We do not want to admit our lack of substance to ourselves and, instead, strive to project an image of completeness, or self-sufficiency. The paradox is that, to the extent that we succumb to this urge, we are estranged from ourselves and are not real. Our narcissism requires that we keep the truth about ourselves at bay.[5, p. 48]

But succumb to that longing for self-sufficiency, power, and completeness many health professionals do. Narcissism offers a model of the self that presumably enables its adherents to keep from falling apart, but with a modus vivendi that invites frustration and unhappiness.

What the individual gains in professional confidence from his attachment to a false self, he loses in warmth, empathy, feeling loved and supported, and relational authenticity. There is a striking correlation in all of this with certain clinical observations made by the great British analyst Donald Winnicott. Epstein quotes Winnicott's remarks on how the false self "is a primitive form of self-sufficiency in the absence of nurture," a strategy of "compliance" that permits the person to survive while hiding out from the unsympathetic parental environment.[6, p. 53] This absent nurturing and sympathy recalls our earlier discussion of the training of the medical intern or resident, wherein he often feels overwhelmed and abjectly alone, yet also feels that a request for help is a sign of weakness. Eric Marcus, whom I mentioned in a previous chapter, conducted research on medical students' dreams and found that a common nightmare of first-year interns was their treating a patient who is rapidly deteriorating. But in the dream, the intern is terrifyingly alone in the emergency or operating room with not a soul to be found anywhere.[7]

The attractive coherence that the narcissistic self offers, the dogged suppression yet occasional protrusion of highly conflicted and painful feelings, and a dedication to the false self's unattainable perfectionism reflect the advanced medical narcissist's pathology: that his or her underlying sense of incompleteness and vulnerability must be remedied. Herein lies the narcissist's ultimate longing. It is why Narcissus could not leave his reflection in the pool even though he knew it spelled his doom, and it explains the last axiom of Hedberg's 12 Step Program described in Chapter 3: We continue to repeat behaviors that are reactions to what we most fear. Epstein quotes Freud's remarking that, "The patient does not remember anything of what he has forgotten and repressed, but acts it out ... He reproduces it not as a memory but as an action; he repeats it, without, of course, knowing that he is repeating it."[8, p. 182] Unable to deal with those fears directly, we opt for the psychological musculature and armor that narcissism offers and then observe the evolution of the self-contained, self-preoccupied, arrogant, and emotionally unavailable medical narcissist.

Given this individual's self-formation, the appearance of serious, harm-causing medical error is therefore not only unsettling; *if acknowledged and reflected upon too deeply, it is an invitation to madness.* In his book, *The Search for the Real Self,* James Masterson speaks of the "Six Horsemen of the Psychical Apocalypse": depression, panic, rage, guilt, helplessness, and emptiness.[9] Medical error throws open the doors of the apocalyptic stables. These reactions are precisely the ones commonly reported in the literature on medical error. And while they indeed exemplify a dedicated health professional, they also characterize the very vulnerabilities his or her narcissism is meant to protect. Let us explore this phenomenon more deeply.

Longings

Epstein quotes the third Zen patriarch Seng-tsan's lesson that, "the greatest source of human anxiety is the experience of nonperfection. Only through the recognition of perfection as a fantasy can such insecurity be overcome; only then can one live 'without anxiety about non-perfection.'"[10, p. 86]

The perfectionist model is immensely familiar in healthcare education and training, but we should pause to reflect on its connotations and associations. Not only does "perfection" token cognitive and behavioral errorlessness and faultlessness, but it also suggests transcendent specialness and superiority, absolute rationality, immortality, indeed, divinity. The false, narcissistic self resonates with these images and the feelings they evoke. Unhealthy narcissists believe that when they ultimately merge with their perfectionistic fantasy, they attain the security, fixedness, lovability, and permanence that perfection promises. The unhealthily narcissistic health professional's longings seem related. Psychoanalysts like to point out how this individual's dedication to eradicating disease, overcoming disability, restoring function, and prolonging life suggests considerable resistance to the reality of life's naturally entropic course, and that such a person must therefore balk at humbling him- or herself before the altar of biophysiological deterioration. And cannot one say that fabricating the false self—with its architecture of solidity, self-control, smugness, and confidence—is the very antithesis of what we know the real self to be and experience: a self that is always in movement and flux; that is frequently bewildered if not profoundly anxious in the face of life's unpredictability; that can usually exert little if any control over the things that matter most in life; that can rarely be certain about anything really important; and whose body is ever so gradually breaking down on its journey toward nonbeing?

Medical error is one of those phenomena that unlocks the vault wherein these fears are normally kept at bay. Indeed, even when we manage error disclosure truthfully and honestly, we might resist that additional step of learning the deepest lessons about the professional self that medical error can teach. That analysis is valuable indeed because I believe it leads to a sacred place: to the psyche of the healer.

The Healer

Clinical health professionals, as opposed to their research counterparts, spend much of their lives reacting, often frantically, to patient care situations. Managed care makes it even more difficult for professionals to be quietly reflective or ruminative, so it is no wonder that many health providers have trouble with listening and silence. Given the stress that so often accompanies the delivery of healthcare, many professionals are understandably anxious about and keen to control the process and content of patient care.

Of course, patients often like it just that way. Despite the rhetoric of the last three decades that champions patient empowerment and informational transparency, it is probably safe to say that many if not most patients unhesitatingly place themselves in their health providers' hands, sit or lie back, and hope for the very best.

Consequently, while I made a case in Chapter 2 for understanding the disclosure of medical error according to the contractual nature of the patient-professional relationship, in reality, that contract is hardly between equal parties. After all, one of them is sick, vulnerable, and relatively uninformed while the other is well, capable, and skillful. The patient hopes to pay for services competently rendered and that yield a superlative outcome, which is often exactly what the service provider gives the patient significant reason to believe will happen.[11]

When a harm-causing medical error occurs, the receiver of services may feel betrayed while the provider may feel like a fraud. This makes the disclosure of error all the more anguishing: The provider must confess his incompetence, which he assumes will trigger the patient's bitterness toward him. By admitting the error to him or herself and to the harmed party as well, the professional must not only withstand the recriminations of his or her conscience but also the harmed party's rage and sadness. How, in such a situation, is the professional supposed to psychologically tolerate such anguish?

Over the years, I have read and thought about the psychological formation of the healthcare professional we might identify as a "healer." I have come to the conclusion that this is a person whose pre-eminent skill consists in using the patient-provider *relationship* therapeutically. Not only able to implement a course of treatment that results in a relatively favorable clinical outcome, the healer is also able to impress the patient with his or her clinical concern and commitment and deeply enjoin the patient, especially on an unconscious level, in that effort. The healer has the remarkable ability to make the patient feel that the patient is the only person in the world who matters. The healer also projects a kind of vitality to the patient, even when there may be reason to believe that the patient's recovery is hopeless. Yet, the healer is able to communicate a clinical expectation to the patient that, no matter how sad or disagreeable, is frequently accepted by the patient with equanimity, grace, and courage.[12] How does that occur?

One reason it occurs, I believe, is because the healer has become aware of whatever unhealthy narcissism he or she may have once harbored and has largely extinguished it. Authentic humility is the polar opposite of narcissism. Just as humiliation in the face of suffering is the first of the Buddha's Four Noble Truths, cultivating humility is the first of the healer's virtues.

The healer acquires his humility by learning to give up his deepest, narcissistic longings because he comes to realize that their contents can never be secured. He learns his humility by becoming convinced of the inevitable frustration inherent in his search for omniscience, absolute certainty, control, categorical respect from others, hedonic satisfaction, and perfect security. He lives the truth that, "One does not err by perceiving, one errs by clinging."[13, p. 157] Perhaps this is why we tend to associate the image of a healer with that of an older person. The healer has learned to be comfortable with the discomfort of uncertainty, impermanence, and, especially, the eventuality of his or her nonbeing.

Because he gives up his narcissistic cravings, the healer is able to realize three things. The first is that he can be content in the moment and use and enjoy its fullness and amplitude to pay "bare attention" to what is happening. With patients, he or she can, as Freud encouraged, "withhold all conscious influences from his capacity to attend, and give himself over completely to his 'unconscious memory.' "[14, pp. 114–115] In that vein, Bernard Lown observes that 50 years of clinical practice led him to:

> …focus more on the interstices between words, on meanings imbedded in pauses, on inflections, on words that emerge haltingly. Silence usually communicates essence. One learns to decipher an unspoken subtext. Intuition is sharpened, enabling me to grasp a new order of complexity, to absorb the subliminal and integrate it almost instantly into a gestalt embodying the true other.[15, p. 20]

The "gestalt embodying the true other" is the primary clinical dividend that the healer's attending-listening-being practice of bare attention provides. By categorically attending to the patient, the meanings that emerge are those of Lown's "true other" and are not fabricated, manipulated, or distorted by the physician's directiveness. By de-centering himself, the healer permits the other's self to emerge. By employing bare attention, the healer silences those elements of his own experience that "remain available for narcissistic recruitment."[16, p. 134] The healer exemplifies the pure attention of the famous Japanese haiku:

The old pond.

A frog jumps in.

Plop![17, p. 113]

The second characteristic of the healer's art is that having traded the narcissistic attraction of permanence for an appreciation of experience's subjective flow, the healer uses narrative to communicate with the patient. The healer knows that the language of science smacks of solidity and reality, but the healer also knows that patients are largely disinterested in that language because they take the professional's mastery of it for granted. On the other hand, the healer understands and respects how narcissistic patients are themselves because their welfare is at stake. So, the healer uses the language of stories and narrative because it is not only more comprehensible and memorable to the patient, but its flow, drama, and event-like character better resonate with the patient's life experience.[18]

The third characteristic of the healer is the ability to empathize. The healer becomes "impartial, open, nonjudgmental, interested, patient, fearless, and impersonal."[19, p. 126] Nonjudgmental and impersonal mean that healers initially resist imposing their evaluations and labels on what they perceive, and instead seek out and study the patient's experiences more deeply. This allows the substance of the patient's experience to emerge more naturally and contextually as facilitated by the relational environment that the healer cultivates.[20]

This last feature, of course, stands in marked contrast to the pathological reactivity of many medical professionals—especially their feeling pressured to respond immediately to what they see and hear for fear they will otherwise feel inept, helpless, or useless. As such, the healer is to be doubly congratulated: first, for his or her insight and stamina to explore and overcome those narcissistic temptations that are prefigured in medical training and practice, and second, for not succumbing to the expediency of narcissism in patient care, with all the dismissive derivatives that attach to it such as lecturing, blaming, sermonizing, threatening, and dismissing.

It is noteworthy how virtually all psychological theories on the etiology of narcissism posit that life begins in a state of narcissistic bliss where all our needs are automatically accommodated.[21] We then carry that expectation into our earliest infancy, where that immediate satisfaction of our needs ends and where we must learn to tolerate frustration and disappointment. No matter how much they might differ, psychological theories largely agree that the narcissist's pathology consists in his or her inability to halt a craving for a permanent return to that all too brief, Garden of Eden state of perfection. The unhealthy narcissist cannot tolerate disappointment, especially when his or her feelings of adequacy are at stake, and rages when such frustrations occur.[22] The healer, however, learns the rather painful truth that life simply does not offer that kind of happiness and satiety and, I believe, communicates that through his own projections to the often very narcissistic patient.

Just as rocks don't swim and pigs don't fly, life doesn't offer the endless stream of mirroring experiences the narcissist craves. When the narcissist deeply realizes and absorbs this truth, he might, like Narcissus, feel immense grief, forlornness, hollowness, and depression. But healers opt for a different course. They manage to locate themselves in a world where a non-narcissistic kind of perfection exists and where:

> [A]ll the creative possibilities of the universe are to be found … It is the innate ability of each of us to … behave with extreme dignity, to conduct our business in a righteous manner, and to channel an endless stream of life enhancing ideas and celebratory sounds for the upliftment of mankind … A most worthy goal is to live one's life and perform all of one's duties living in and from this inner space. "Out of the fullness of this presence of mind, disturbed by no ulterior motive, the artist who is released from all attachment must practice his art." [23, p. 77]

But, alas, in practicing that art, even the healer makes mistakes and errors. What might his or her reaction be to the anguish that such experiences cause?

Errors and Humility

The individual who achieves the kind of enlightenment learned from authentic humility will feel an immense sadness from error. Yet, his or her primary reaction will not, I think, be one of disgrace because empathy for the harmed party directs attention away from his or her own self-preoccupation.[24] Embarrassment betrays our narcissistic longings. If one can abandon that baggage, however, one's feelings will instead take the form of a devoted attention to those who are suffering. The healer feels a profound debt to those who were harmed and is grieved by the possibility, especially in instances of catastrophic error, that the debt might never be eradicated. But without the encumbrance of embarrassment, the healer's empathy and sorrow for the harmed party is all the more pure.

Without the self-referentiality of embarrassment, the healer does not feel an incapacitating blow to his or her adequacy despite the error's horrific effects. Rather, the healer accepts his or her imperfections and recognizes that, as much as one tries to prevent them, harm-causing errors will occur. What the healer will do, however, is contain whatever professional anger wells up in the midst of an error investigation. The healer recalls the relativity of blame: how easy it is to blame others, how hard to direct that blame toward oneself, and how unjust the blaming might ultimately turn out to be.

The healer also recognizes that whatever vengefulness and fury the harmed parties exhibit are valid expressions of their wounded selves. And while the healer grieves with them over their having been wronged, he or she understands that their hatred and destructive impulses derive from their perfectly appropriate belief that this error should not have occurred. The healer hopes that an empathic approach will succeed in modulating the harmed party's initial feelings of rage into feelings of grief, sorrow, and, perhaps, acceptance.[25]

The healer realizes that while harm-causing error tokens an unallowable wrong and thus merits a justice response, the essential character of serious harm-causing error is ultimately that of tragedy—a tragedy wherein a group of human beings, meeting in the midst of hard-to-imagine complexities and contingencies, sought a much-desired outcome but experienced a great misfortune. While healers cannot control how others will absorb that tragedy, their own sense of self remains relatively intact. Because they have long given up an interest in cultivating a narcissistic-like professional aura, healers are not incapacitated by error. Therein lies the essence of their healthy pride: the satisfaction in healing done for its own sake, not for whatever respect, admiration, or attention it brings. Alternatively, the healthcare professional who develops an intense need for respect or attention is at immense psychological risk when an unanticipated outcome appears.

Without these narcissistically embedded self-preoccupations, the healer can be completely present to those who were harmed. He or she acknowledges their right to information, desists from finding fault anywhere—so that if asked where fault might lie, he or she will only remark that "we were all to blame"—and may indeed ask for forgiveness. The request for forgiveness stems from the healer's only vestige of narcissism: namely, that the healer needs to be forgiven for subjecting another human being to risk and then failing to reasonably protect the other from whatever harm materialized. Even from one who learned humility, this stands as the great narcissistic paradox of the healer: that practicing his or her art inevitably requires a kind of hubris or even bravado that exposes others to serious risk and danger. If the healer chides himself or herself for anything, it will be that. And if fury is vented at the healer, he or she absorbs and contains it because the healer recognizes that his or her audacity, although well-intended, has caused others sadness and pain. So, too, the healer understands forgiveness as a permission from the harmed party that he or she can go on.

As healers contain their narcissism in the midst of error disclosure, so there is a good probability that the narcissism of the harmed parties will be likewise contained. Despite the harmed party's natural desire to avenge the wrong, the healer's humility will shear that wrongdoing of the further insult that a "densely self-conscious" approach to error disclosure might cause. Impressed with the healer's self-effacement and singular commitment to them, the harmed individual's rage has nowhere to go. Hence, there is a good chance it will dim and leave only sadness in its wake.[26]

The impossibility of realizing closure in many instances of harm-causing error is, perhaps, its most anguishing characteristic. Neither an error admission, apology, explanation, counseling, or large malpractice award can ever right the damage a single disastrous error can cause. But healers know that life does not operate according to a banker's ledger of debits and credits, and an insistence that it does is a prescription for further suffering. The kind of insurance against unhappiness that the narcissist seeks throughout his or her life is simply unavailable—which perhaps explains why the healer's wisdom and persona sometimes seem tinged with a quiet, almost reverential sadness. Healers know that perfect happiness, justice, or satisfaction are utterly unattainable and perhaps cannot help feeling saddened by that realization, as well as feeling sadness for those who doggedly pursue those fantasies. As Oscar Wilde observed in a somber moment: "Where there is sorrow, there is holy ground."[27, p. 676]

The healer's humility allows him or her to react both empathically to the error and then to move on. Humility enables healers to do what any successful psychological intervention does for the unwell: It enables the sufferer to understand and feel the experience *differently*.[28] This means that healers will proceed through life without self-pity or rage or a burning need to seek relief from the anguish of their errors. Instead, the healer will proceed in a way that affirms life, that reinforces his or her feeling good by doing good, and that recognizes the inevitability and universality of human suffering and error.

In his lovely book, *The Heart Aroused*, David Whyte tells the story of meeting three barefoot and shoddy pilgrims near the Tibetan border of Nepal.[29] The three turn out to be middle-class university professors who, at the age of 50, decide to follow a popular Indian tradition: They leave their jobs, go on a long sabbatical, and reflect on their lives. They walk 800 miles to visit a sacred temple and upon arriving at the holy place they bow, say a prayer, walk three times around the temple, and abruptly leave. Whyte recalls, "I watched them walking down that long valley toward the plains and felt for the first time the central importance of the *journey* itself."[30, p. 209]

Was theirs an object lesson on how life largely consists of what happens *between* our moments of ecstasy and despondency? Realize that the narcissist is most affected by life's zeniths and nadirs, singularly devoting himself to merging with the former, and being utterly uncomprehending and enraged by an encounter with the latter. The healer, on the other hand, knows that most of life is neither one nor the other but, as captured in these lines from the poet Rilke:

> ... the rest between two notes,
>
> Which are somehow always in discord
>
> because death's note wants to climb over—
>
> but in the dark interval, reconciled,
>
> They stay there trembling.
>
> And the song goes on, beautiful.[31, p. 241]

The Narcissus

Perhaps the narcissus flower, as Thomas Moore points out, represents the ultimate triumph of Narcissus's tragedy. There are thousands of varieties of narcissi, just as there are thousands of different kinds of narcissists. The flower has its season; it can only be according to its nature; and its life above the earth is relatively short. But it is a perennial, with a deep root system so that new flowers emerge in the Spring.[32] Its power and vigor, then, lie not in what we see above the surface but beneath it. Therein lies its real solidity and permanence—and indeed, its darkness, dirtiness, even ugliness. Even when the flower reappears in the Spring and reclaims its place above the surface, it will in its maturity incline its petals not toward the sun, but toward the earth. As a flower, it cannot know itself or be aware of its beauty. It cannot pursue perfection or defend itself from assault. It can only be. And in its quiet and brief life, it is admired by everyone.

Whatever beauty and health the flower enjoys depend on how hospitable and nurturing its environment is. Let us hope, then, that our healer-educators can help those they teach to develop healthy roots. Let us hope these young, aspiring professionals will have had their beginnings in nourishing environments where they were raised by good-enough parents; that they are taught the art of medicine by good-enough instructors; and that they will develop the equanimity to weather the storms of their lives as well as the beautiful, sunshiny days. Most importantly, let us hope that our healing and teaching environments will help all who stumble upon their image in the pond and are dazzled by what they see to understand that life does not offer real fulfillment to those who relentlessly pursue their imagined, ideal selves, but rather to those who seek to be one with others:

> Though the reflection in the pool
> Often swims before our eyes:
> Know the image.
>
> Only in the dual realm
> do voices become
> eternal and mild.[33, p.75]

(Rilke, Sonnets to Orpheus)

References

1. Gelb, Michael J. *Discover Your Genius*. New York: HarperCollins, 2002.

2. Epstein, Mark. *thoughts without a thinker*. New York: Basic Books, 1995.

3. Millon, Theodore. *Disorder of Personality: DSM-IV and Beyond*. New York: John Wiley & Sons, Inc., 1996, pp. 393–427.

4. Epstein, 1995.

5. Epstein, 1995.

6. Epstein, 1995.

7. Marcus, Eric. "Empathy, humanism, and the professionalization process of medical education." *Academic Medicine*. 74(11):1211–1215, 1999.

8. Epstein, 1995.

9. Masterson, James F. *The Search for the Real Self*. New York: The Free Press, 1988, p. 61.

10. Epstein, 1995.

11. Levinson, Wendy, and Chaumeton, Nigel. "Communication between surgeons and patients in routine office visits." *Surgery*. 125(2):127–134, 1999.

12. Lown, Bernard. *The Lost Art of Healing: Practicing Compassion in Medicine.* New York: Ballantine Books, 1999.

13. Epstein, 1995.

14. Lown, 1999.

15. Lown, 1999.

16. Epstein, 1995.

17. Epstein, 1995.

18. Buckman, Robert, and Kason, Yvonne. *How to Break Bad News.* Baltimore, MD: The Johns Hopkins University Press, 1992.

19. Epstein, 1995.

20. Lown, 1999.

21. Epstein, 1995.

22. Masterson, 1988.

23. Werner, Kenny. *Effortless Mastery.* New Albany, IN: Jamey Aebersold Jazz, Inc., 1996.

24. Exline, Julie Juola, and Baumeister, Roy F. "Expressing forgiveness and repentance." In Michael McCullough, Kenneth Pargament, and Carl Thoresen, eds. *Forgiveness: Theory, Research, and Practice*, New York: The Guilford Press, 2000, pp. 133–157.

25. Exline and Baumeister, 2000.

26. Exline and Baumeister, 2000.

27. Wilde, Oscar. *De Profundis.* Quoted in Bartlett, John. Familiar Quotations, 15th edition. Boston, MA: Little, Brown and Company, 1980.

28. Epstein, 1995.

29. Whyte, David. *The Heart Aroused.* New York: Currency/Doubleday, 1996.

30. Whyte, 1996.

31. Rilke, Rainer Maria. The poem is translated by Robert Bly and quoted in Whyte, David, 1996.

32. See the following websites: http://www.angelfire.com/journal2/flowers/d.html; http://www.flowers.org.uk/flowers/facts/k-r/narcissus.htm; http://www.about-flowers.org/thepoetsdaffo xfg.htm; http://www.cyberkisses.com/Scenery/flowerlegend.html.

33. Rilke, Rainer Maria. *Sonnets to Orpheus.* The poem is translated by Robert Whyte and quoted in Whyte, 1996.

Error Rationalization and the Somatically Marking Brain

Introduction

This appendix is included for the sake of adding a third model of rationalization to the two that are presented in Chapter 2. The discussion that follows, however, is highly speculative as it relies on certain fairly recent neuroscientific findings but reconstructs them in a way that is very different from the research that originated them. The model is nevertheless presented because it suggests a *neurobiological* basis for rationalization that lends further credibility to Goleman's model of selective attention. Moreover, the model gives some suggestions as to how the narcissism construct discussed in Chapter 3 and Appendix 2 might be understood neurobiologically.

Emotional Ethics

A very prominent strain of moral philosophy that reaches its apotheosis in Kant but originates at least with Plato insists that moral deliberation ought to be a purely rational activity wherein feelings, emotions, passions, and self-interest play no substantive role. On this view, feelings and emotions contaminate a person's ability to determine what is "universally" (for Kantians) or "really" (for Platonists) right or good. This sensibility permeates much of classical moral philosophy: Philosophers such as Plato and Kant argue that the subjective and especially emotional trappings of ethical life—for example, a person's interest in self-preservation or the importance attached to an individual's drives, wants, personal preferences, and needs—distracts from the objective content of moral behavior, that is, duties and obligations as they might be *rationally* deduced, inferred, or determined.[1]

Without addressing the various arguments that repudiate the role of emotions and feelings in moral reasoning, it is worth pointing out that the normal brain's willful banishment of emotions and feelings from moral deliberation (or any kind of deliberation for that matter) is now known to be a neurological impossibility. Contemporary neuroscientific research makes it abundantly clear that not only are consciousness and emotions inseparable, but that when the two are disconnected—such as occurs in instances of brain cancer or brain trauma—practical reasoning becomes markedly dysfunctional.[2]

To appreciate the neurobiological role of the emotions in the context of human cognition, start with the fact that the brain evolved from the spinal cord up. First to evolve was the brain stem, then the hypothalamus, thalamus, and the rest of the limbic system, and then the associative cortices and the wraparound neocortex. The intense experiences of anguish accompanying the realization of a medical error as described in Chapter 2 are hardly Kantian "detached reasoning" reactions, but are largely mediated by hypothalamic and other limbic system activations coursing through numerous brain-body structures. These brain events inject a virtual flood of hormones, neurotransmitters, neuropeptides, cytokines, and other neurochemicals into the brain's limbic system, the various sensory and frontal cortices, and the hippocampus situated inside the temporal lobes.[3]

Neuroscientists would say that the marked psychophysical reactions of these anguished health providers upon learning of their errors typify the brain's functional response to extreme stress: When the organism experiences a threat to its welfare, the brain's physiologic responses act to increase the organism's survival probability, such as occurs with increased metabolism, circulation, blood clotting factors, blood pressure, and respiration. Because the brain evolved from the spinal cord up, it is logical to assume that the brain is primordially interested in the body's preservation, due to the fact that the role of the brain stem is to monitor and regulate the body's most basic "vegetative" functions such as thermoregulation, metabolism, and wakefulness. These ancient brain structures are hardly centers of analytical and deliberative reasoning but are triggers and processors of feelings and emotions that communicate with—because they are neurologically hard-wired with—areas of the brain that evolved later and that are more involved in thinking, planning, and calculating (e.g., the orbital frontal cortex, the inferior temporal lobes, and the prefrontal cortex).[4] Indeed although the brain's thalamus receives sensory inputs from the sense organs and then sends these messages to whatever areas of the sensory and frontal cortices that decipher or interpret them, the thalamus simultaneously sends a much faster but cruder message to the amygdala that alerts the body's metabolic processors for the possibility of a fight or flight response. (See Figure A-1.) While the sensory and associational cortices along with the hippocampus inform the amygdala of what is going on milliseconds later, it is immensely revealing that the ancient, emotional centers of the brain want to have a first look at incoming stimuli. Indeed, the brain circuitry linking the emotional processing of the limbic system *to* the analytical and deliberative areas of the frontal cortices is considerably more dense and elaborate than the pathways *from* the frontal cortices to the limbic system.[5] This leads some scholars to opine that the brain's architecture is clearly biased toward emotions affecting reasoning rather than the other way around (although thousands of years from now, when evolution will have changed neurophysiology, the struc-

Figure A-1 *Memory and the Brain's Stress Response*

Sensory Cortex	**Transitional cortex** / Perirhinal cortex / Parahippocampal cortex / Entorhinal cortex
Sensory Thalamus → **Amygdala**	**Hippocampus**
Emotional Stimulus	**Hypothalamus** (Releases CRF or Corticotrophin-releasing factor)
	Pituitary Gland (Releases Adrenocorticotrophic hormone or ACTH)
	Adrenal Cortex (releases cortisol or CORT)

Adapted from Joseph LeDoux, *The Emotional Brain*, p. 241.

tures of these neural pathways might significantly change). This also explains why talk therapy or psychoanalysis take a long time to diminish a person's habituated fears, and why the self-help section of the bookstore does not carry titles like *How You Can Become More Fearful* or *How You Can Increase Your Stress*. Stress, fear, anger, and aggression are ancient, hard-wired, primitive brain functions that do not require cultivation. In the process of its evolution, the brain decided that its best chances of survival lay with a greater reliance on its emotional circuitry than with its purely ratiocinative prowess. As discussed later, that ratiocination would have little survival value without its being coupled with the brain's awesome ability to bio-regulate thinking and reasoning.

Emotions Informing Reason

Antonio Damasio is well known for his book, *Descartes Error*, in which he advances what he calls the "somatic marker hypothesis." The somatic marker hypothesis (SMH) is an attempt to describe how the feeling structures of the brain modulate and "inform" cognition and thinking. In what follows, Damasio's SMH is used as a theoretical element in speculating on the neurology of rationalization.

The SMH is Damasio's attempt to show how the brain imbues its representational contents with importance or salience so that human beings can connect their ideational life with survival-optimizing behaviors. In their most basic form, somatic markers act as an internal preference system that is "inherently biased to avoid pain, seek potential pleasure, and is probably pre-tuned for achieving these goals in social situations."[6, p. 179]

A somatic marker is not a deliberative act but rather the brain's way of *affectively* signaling certain thinking-behaving options as either dangerous or favorable while eliminating others as irrelevant or inefficient. Certain markers or "tokens of salience" appear to be innate as, for example, a newborn's intuitively attending to and searching the facial expressions of his parents and even mimicking their expressions such as sticking out the tongue in response to the parent's doing the same.[7] Although less than an hour old, some newborns display this instinctive reaction, which shows that neonates can attentively target certain objects in their visual and olfactory fields as salient. Already these newborns have the neurological capability to mimic what they perceive, which involves their ability to attend to and physiologically "empathize" with what they are perceiving so as to duplicate it with their own bodies.

While some somatic markers are innate, Damasio contends that most result from socialization and experiential learning. The ability to learn social conventions and ethical rules is made possible by the way the brain affectively marks and conjoins specific cognitions with specific behaviors. Much of the human self is constituted by the nature and development of a person's somatic marking because those markers explain the decisional-behavioral patterns that typify that person as him- or herself. Faculty in the schools of medicine, health, and law know this extremely well even if they might not articulate it in Damasio's terms. Students are typically "impressionable," and much of their learning occurs through enculturation and socialization. Sound moral behavior, then, is facilitated by students finding themselves in morally healthy atmospheres that, per Damasio's model, witness the somatic marking of ethically sound values, attitudes, beliefs, and behaviors. In contrast, consider the neurosurgeon who once told me that when he was in training, he and his fellow residents were explicitly instructed never to disclose an error to a patient and always charge for whatever treatments the patient might require as a result of the error. The physician said, "My supervisor told me that deleting charges might trigger the patient's suspicions that an error happened." Whether or not this physician practiced his supervisor's advice, it clearly made such an impression on him that he could recite the advice years later. It is also an example of the "professional" advice that many physicians receive in training that shapes some of their morally problematic thinking-behavioral responses to the commission of medical error and to other ethically charged situations as well.

Rationalizations as Salienced Representations

Damasio and his colleagues spent a good deal of time considering the probable neural pathways—largely implicating the limbic system, the temporal lobes, the cingulated gyrus, and the prefrontal cortices—by which ideas are prioritized and imbued with salience or value so that coherent decision making can occur. When these pathways are disrupted by disease or injury, the brain subsequently loses its capacity to give salience to its representations; then decision making can become utterly dysfunctional.[8]

Damasio's evidence for the SMH derives from his studies of individuals whose frontal cortices were damaged. While their intelligence and primary emotions remained intact, these persons could not imbue their ideas, representations, or mental images with feelings or emotions as measured by skin conductance tests such as are used in polygraphs. That inability resulted in frankly impaired decision and choice making when these persons were enrolled in penalty-reward type experiments.

In one particular experiment, participants with frontal lobe damage were asked to pick from four decks of cards, and they were monetarily rewarded or penalized without initially knowing why. The decks were arranged, however, so that choosing a card from the first or second decks provided the chooser with either a high reward but at other times an even higher punishment. Choosing a card from the third or fourth decks resulted in a lower reward but at other times an even lower penalty. Normals, or persons with undamaged brains, not only got the hang of the undisclosed rules fairly quickly—that is, choose from decks one and two and you will eventually lose all your money, but choose from decks three and four and you will slowly but surely make money—they manifested a neurophysiological reaction in their card choosings that Damasio used as an evidential linchpin for the SMH. After a significant enough number of choosings from the various decks, whenever the normal would go to choose from decks one and two, he or she would register a significant "peremptory" galvanic skin response, indicating a kind of stress reaction whose severity did not occur when he or she chose from decks three and four. *Frontal lesion patients, however, not only registered no such galvanic response in choosing from decks three and four, but in other experiments they registered no discernible response to emotionally provocative pictorial images of fear and the like, even though they understood the meanings of the pictures.*

The consistency of these findings led Damasio and his colleagues to hypothesize that it was not the case that frontal lesion patients were incapable of primary emotional responses because they registered startle responses to noise and strobe light and displayed appropriate galvanic responses to immediate reward and punishment. Rather, patients with damage to their frontal lobes apparently suffered from memory and attentional deficits that resulted in their inability to "mark" those images or representations such that they can be used in future decision making. These individuals seemed incapable of formulating productive or successful future behaviors from their past experiences. Unlike normals, they showed no anticipatory responses that would indicate that their brains were developing a predictive capacity for negative future outcomes. This "predictive capacity," Damasio reasoned, is essentially the work of somatic markers.

This suggests that the SMH might lend a certain degree of neurobiological support for Goleman's theory of moral attention. Goleman's representations that provoke either moral attentiveness or inattentiveness can be read in Damasio's model as somatically marked images or representations (e.g., as attractive, repellant, or uninteresting representations) that trigger certain behavioral dispositions. Consider the theoretical proximity of Damasio's SMH with Goleman's model of selective attention in this passage from *Descartes Error*:

> [W]hen different somatic markers are juxtaposed to different combinations of images, they modify the way the brain handles them, and thus operate as a bias. The bias might allocate attentional enhancement differently to each component, the consequences being the automated assigning of varied degrees of attention to varied contents, which translates into an uneven landscape.[9, p. 199]

In instances of recognizing harm-causing medical error, it just might be that the somatic accents of the professional's mental landscape of "uneven" images derive from his or her feelings of horror and intense anxiety; additional feelings of terror that contemplating the disclosure of the error might trigger; and the moral disgust that might arise in seriously considering concealment. If the individual believes that his or her professional survival after an honest disclosure of error is improbable and he or she simultaneously experiences significant neurobiological activity mediating a stress reaction, Damasio's model can be extrapolated to suggest that the brain will be progressively inclined to tag "rationalizing representations" *favorably*. As such, those somatic tags favoring rationalization suggest a neurobiological explanation of Goleman's attentional selectivity model: The fact that attention is attracted to or saliences certain images or representations—that is, the rationalized ones—exhibits the organism's way of disposing with the immense psychological discomfort that other representations present, that is, the painful but morally obligatory ones bearing on error disclosure.

Note too that representational salience includes an interpretational act, but in instances of moral rationalization, "interpretation" becomes "distortion." The individual who rationalizes medical error gives salience to certain conceptual features of the error situation that should not have moral sway. But because the organism might fear for its own welfare, the distortion becomes self-serving: By repeatedly recalling the event but modifying, rethinking, reshaping, and re-evaluating it each time, somatic marking shapes the now distorted situation into one that no longer recognizes an error as an error, or an error that causes harm, or as an error that causes harm that is not so bad after all, or as an error that causes dreadful harm but that it is someone else's fault.

Biasing Memory Formation

There is one more neurological finding that might support this process of cognitive or representational distortion. While stress often sharpens attention, neuroscientists now recognize how the pituitary, hypothalamic, and adrenally mediated release of too much steroidal hormone can damage the hippocampus, which is one of the brain's primary memory processors. When the hippocampus is damaged, it is less able to formulate and consolidate accurate memories, prompting Joseph LeDoux to note in his popular book *The Emotional Brain*:

[I]f the hippocampus was only partially affected by the trauma, it may have participated in the formation of a weak and fragmented memory. In such a situation, it may be possible to mentally reconstruct aspects of the experience. Such memories will by necessity involve "filling in the blanks," and the accuracy of the memory will be a function of how much filling in was done and how critical the filled-in parts were to the essence of the memory ... Even memories that are formed with a perfectly well-functioning hippocampus are easily distorted by experiences that occur between the formation of the memory and its retrieval.[10, p. 244]

Although memories are distributed throughout the brain, the hippocampus is crucial in memory formation. As illustrated in Figure A–1, the hippocampus along with the sensory and associational cortices might turn out to be a major culprit in the distortion, confabulation, or rationalization of medical error—or any moral dilemma whose anxiety-provoking nature is intolerable—because one of its chief roles is to regulate the amount of adrenal steroid hormone (called cort or cortisol) that goes into the body and then back to the brain. In conjunction with other neural networks, especially the frontal cortices, the hippocampus can co-opt whatever moral inclinations encourage moral behaviors by re-representing or misremembering the moral dilemma in such a way that the "final and official" version of what happened is singularly self-serving. Because one role of the hippocampus is to modulate the amount of cortisol being released into the body—especially as that cortisol release is also triggered by the amygdala—the brain might cleverly figure out a way to relieve anxiety by reconstructing the precipitating stimulus, that is, the error event, so that the dilemma disappears along with its associated trauma. In conjunction with a hippocampus-impaired memory consolidation, the somatic marker phenomenon might therefore work to draw attention to those representations or images that the self deems to be in its best interest, even if the brain has to fabricate them.

Limitations of the SMH for the Explanation of Moral Rationalization

Some comment is in order regarding the speculations and guesswork that the neurobiological model described here presents in explaining moral rationalization.

First of all, there are no hard data that explicitly inform a neurological theory of rationalization or self-deception. Damasio's SMH is, instead, an attempt to explain how certain of the brain's representations take on significance and importance so that cognition has coherence and decision making enhances the probability of survival. Damasio certainly does not pose the SMH as a possible model to explain moral rationalization or even cognitive distortion. What he does is depict the SMH as a positive, indeed indispensable, attribute for effective cognitive functioning. Nevertheless, there is room to wonder whether the SMH might also explain how moral reasoning and moral behavior are compromised in rationalization.

Second, the SMH derives from studies of individuals with damaged frontal cortices. Because these individuals are unable to activate bio-regulatory neural networks that inform the consequences of their decisions or responses in an effective way, these individuals wind up making disastrous decisions. Damasio infers from this that normals possess healthy bio-regulatory capacity and that without it, cognitive life would be in shambles. But this only reemphasizes the speculative nature of using the SMH as an explanatory vehicle for rationalization. In rationalizing medical error, the rationalizers have undamaged brains. Moreover, because it is quite possible that moral rationalization might be subserved by neural pathways that are quite distinct from those utilized in "normal" somatic marking, using the SMH to explain rationalization might well turn out to be a flight of fancy.

Third, the SMH and many other studies of the brain's emotional and cognitive processing examine rather rudimentary brain activity, such as how the brain processes simple stimuli such as a tone or a photograph of a person's face. The "thinking" that is being examined is therefore about very basic acts of recognition (e.g., "That's a siren," or "That's a picture of an angry person").[11] It is therefore rather far from theories about how sentences that mix declarative with emotional content such as, "Well, perhaps the medical error that killed Mr. Jones was a blessing in disguise," are processed in the brain. It is even more of a stretch to confidently propose that neural networks subserve thinking about a densely elaborate medical situation, such as a scenario that might or might not have admitted questionable healthcare, or a scenario wherein it is uncertain whether an error caused harm because any number of variables might have affected the patient's outcome. Indeed, in such scenarios, resistance to error disclosure might not be motivated by rationalizing at all but by an honest struggle to determine how clinical facts and moral obligations intersect.

Fourth, it is necessary to admit that the act of rationalization is probably many steps removed from the kinds of immediate decisions or cognitive acts in which Damasio's research participants engaged. For them, the somatic marker was directly tagged to immediate choices for which they were rewarded or punished in various experiments involving decision making. The kind of rationalization activities described here, though, are often reiterated interpretations, that is, repeated recollections that are markedly removed from the original event that precipitated the professional's emotional discomfort. Do entirely different neural mechanisms, then, subserve the much more elaborate "interpretational" process that winds up distorting a person's moral thinking?

And that question brings up a fifth problem: It becomes somewhat unclear just what is being rationalized and thus somatically marked in this usurpation of Damasio's SMH model. Is the original "experience" of the error primarily distorted in the rationalization, as speculated in remarking on the possibility of hippocampal dysfunction resulting from an excessive stress response? Or does the memory of the original experience remain essentially intact and thus neurologically unchanged, but what changes is the linguistic representation of it? If the latter, what is the relationship between the bare, unarticulated, or "felt" meaning embodied in the original experience of the error situation, which is more akin to the kinds of experiences that Damasio studied in developing the SMH, versus the "lingua form" or sentential meaning that ultimately becomes the rationalization as described? With what certainty can it be professed that the neural mechanisms that mediate the *interpretational trajectory of rationalization*—moving from an unadorned, objective account of what happened, to the more elaborate embroidery of the rationalization itself—are the same as the neural mechanisms described in the SMH? The point here is that the movement from a body state registered by a manifestly unpleasant emotional reaction to the linguistic representation of a moral rationalization is a very long one.

These criticisms are offered not because they might be fatal to the argument that links the SMH to moral rationalization but rather to illustrate the degree of conjecture that is implicit in wondering about the neural substrates of rationalizing. Nevertheless, while it would not be surprising if future neuroscientific investigation implicates a neurological model of moral rationalization that is entirely different from Damasio's SMH, it would be immensely surprising if that model implicates a conceptual schema of rationalization that contrasts sharply with what has been explored here: namely, the cognitive interplay between (in)attention and ideational salience. Rationalization results in the weaker argument defeating the stronger and thus requires a distortion in moral valuing. That valuing, however, is nothing other than the brain ascribing salience to certain of its contents in such a way that psychological and moral agitation is reduced or resolved. It appears, then, that a person's narcissistically based survival instincts, the maintenance of a coherent self-image as a moral individual, and the developmental history of moral sensibilities as expressed by a storehouse of representational saliences will continue to be crucial explanatory elements of any account of rationalization. Although it might turn out that a neural model quite different from Damasio's SMH will have greater explanatory power for comprehending rationalization, it is safe to say it will nevertheless be one that, like the SMH, makes an attempt to explain representational salience.

References

1. Wilson, James Q. *The Moral Sense*. New York: The Free Press, 1993, pp. 191–221.
2. Damasio, Antonio R. *Descartes' Error: Emotion, Reason, and the Human Brain*. New York: Avon Books, 1994.
3. LeDoux, Joseph. *The Emotional Brain*. New York: Simon & Schuster, 1998.
4. LeDoux, 1998.
5. LeDoux, 1998.
6. Damasio, 1994.

7. Churchland, Patricia Smith. *Brain-Wise*. Cambridge, Mass: MIT Press, 2002, pp. 100–102.

8. Damasio, 1994.

9. Damasio, 1994.

10. LeDoux, 1998.

11. Churchland, 2002.

Becoming
a Narcissist

Introduction

This appendix briefly discusses some of the more technical, especially etiological, aspects of pathological narcissism as they appear in the psychoanalytic literature. Beginning with an interpretation of the myth of Narcissus, what follows identifies certain critical moments in an individual's psychological development that can affect whether his or her narcissism proceeds in a healthy or an unhealthy direction. As noted in Chapter 3, however, the narcissistic character disorder that is most familiar in the literature is not typical of the one I am claiming is found in medicine. It is nevertheless offered here for the sake of readers who are interested in learning more about how the pathological narcissist is psychoanalytically understood.

The Myth of Narcissus

The story of Narcissus is one of the most familiar Greco-Roman myths. Narcissus appears in Ovid's *Metamorphoses* as an emotionally distant youth who, one day, catches sight of his reflection in a pond.[1] His initial delight and then intoxication with his image turns fatal. Hopelessly attached to his reflection, Narcissus pines away beside the pool and dies. Like all people who are consumed by themselves, Narcissus elicits little of our sympathy. A closer reading of Ovid's story, however, might give pause.

First of all, Narcissus was born from the river God Cephisus's rape of his "water-lady" mother, Liriope. The psychotherapist Thomas Moore underlines this circumstance of Narcissus's conception as signifying that Narcissus inherits a persona that is watery, slippery, and lacking in substance.[2] The way others are attracted to Narcissus's beauty and the way they express their affections for him make him feel special and superior. But Narcissus has "little feeling for either boys or girls," and he refuses to place his feelings, especially his affections, in the hands of others. Narcissus attracts everyone, plays with their feelings, and then rejects them. Realizing that Narcissus will never return his affection, a spurned lover curses Narcissus saying, "O may he love himself alone and yet fail in that great love," which the goddess Nemesis hears and makes come true.

With this curse upon him, Narcissus stumbles upon the pool in the depths of the forest and bends over it to slake his thirst. He sees his image reflected in the water and is enchanted although he has no idea that he is looking at himself. So great is Narcissus's lack of self-awareness that he tries to embrace and kiss the image but:

> What he had tried to hold resided nowhere,
>
> For had he turned away, it fell to nothing:
>
> His love was cursed.

Every attempt Narcissus makes to merge with the beautiful figure in the pool fails. He cannot understand why this lovely object at one moment seems as attracted to him as he is to it, only to have it disappear into nothing the next, until he finally realizes that "I am what I long for." As he comes to know himself, Narcissus finds that his self-love cannot sustain him. He has come to "look deeply" into himself but the realization is traumatic, recalling the prophecy of the blind seer Tiresias who predicted that Narcissus could survive into old age only if he defied the oracle and *never* came to know himself. As Tiresias foresaw, Narcissus would be unable to use his self-knowledge so as to rise above it. Narcissus cannot understand that there might be more richness to life than his self-absorption. So, he succumbs to his "image," dies beside the pool, and is swallowed up by the earth. Later at that spot, the beautiful flower narcissus springs up—a gesture, perhaps, of the gods' sympathy.

Water is the central metaphor of the Narcissus myth. Narcissus is conceived in it; his personality is defined by it; it offers him his greatest delight; he comes to self-knowledge through it; and, curiously, it offers him a chance for redemption if only he can somehow understand that the "reflection" he sees is but a partial, watery representation of who he really is. The image in the pool is not the real Narcissus, but a shallow, on-the-surface representation that is exquisitely fragile and evanescent. Toss a stone into the water and the image shatters.[3]

Because Narcissus cannot overcome his fascination and involvement with his self-image, his real self begins to shrivel and die. Why? Because as any psychologist will point out, the common belief that narcissists love themselves excessively distracts from their real pathology. The primary problem among narcissists is that they are unable to love themselves or others in a healthy way.[4] As will be shown, pathological narcissists can only love others who either constantly affirm their grandiose self-image or whom the narcissist extravagantly and unrealistically idealizes. At bottom, narcissists are dysfunctional lovers. They are either so assured of their special place in the universe that they have no feelings or interest in others, or they are so anxious about their lovability that their personal agenda and self-idealization become the driving, signal forces of their lives. Either way, they are headed toward personal and interrelational distress.

A Healthy Regard for Otherness

Heinz Kohut and Otto Kernberg, the twentieth century's pre-eminent theorists on the narcissistic personality disorder, pointed out that healthy psychological development witnesses not only the capacity to feel ample, fulfilled, whole, even grandiose, but it also includes a capacity to regard others in a way that their otherness is acknowledged and appreciated.[5] Kernberg and Kohut theorized that this healthy psychological development consists, among other things, of the child's healthily developing both "mirroring" and "idealizing" transferences.[6] Mirroring transferences occur when the child understands and feels elated that the other—typically and most importantly his parent—is acknowledging and positively affirming his being. The mythical Narcissus experienced this transference when he thought the reflection in the pond was adoring him. Children anticipate these transferences when they scream to their parents, "Mommy! Daddy! Watch me! Watch me!" Idealizing transferences occur when the individual understands an object—be it a person or experience like the practice of medicine—as sweeping, magnificent, and awesome and then proceeds to identify with it, saying, in effect, "*That* is what I want to be, what I want to devote myself to because it is so wonderful." Just so, Narcissus's idealizing perception of the intoxicatingly beautiful image in the pond witnessed his trying to embrace it and merge his being with it.

Notice that powerful mirroring and idealizing transferences are by nature intoxicating, blissful, and all-encompassing. If life consisted of nothing but these moments, everyone would be outrageously happy creatures. But infants quickly learn that life is not a continuous stream of mirroring and self-identifying idealizations. The hope for mirroring transferences is painfully disappointed by the parent who lets the child know in no uncertain terms how much he or she disapproves of the child's behavior; likewise, the child's deeply committed emotional trust and investment in certain people and objects is often disappointed when they turn out to be not nearly as perfect, loving, or ideal as they first (transferentially) appeared.[7]

The child's natural responses to such disappointments are sadness, anger, and rage to which, in Donald Winnicott's precious phrase, the "good enough mother" will respond with emotional comfort and support.[8] This good enough parent will use the child's experience to help the child develop a set of realistic anticipations and beliefs about his or her world that will enable the child to preserve his or her psychological equilibrium in the face of disappointment. The good enough parent will especially know how to enable the child to internalize and cope with his or her disappointment so that he or she can evolve a self-formation that recognizes and manages life's frustrations in a mature rather than infantile way. With appropriate but not oppressive, overly protective, manipulative, or excessive love and attention—thus, he or she is good "enough"—this parent will provide a healthy psychological environment whereby the child can develop what Winnicott and the ego-psychology movement dub healthy or mature "self-object" relations.[9] Put simply, healthy or mature self-object relations imply that one's feelings and behaviors are regulated by a pragmatically reliable understanding of the boundaries and limits that characterize one's relationships, such that he or she does not consistently harbor or confabulate unrealistic expectations of people and things; is not excessively pre-occupied with worries over their successes or failures; is not emotionally devastated when an anticipation is dashed; and can recover from life's more serious disappointments.

Psychologists like to describe all this as the individual's "well integrated subject-object representations" whereby the individual understands that the object as well as he or she admits *both* positive and negative characteristics.[10] The well-integrated ego takes all this in stride. He or she has no trouble accepting the old adage "You're not as good as your last victory nor as bad as your last defeat." The pathological narcissist, on the other hand, never develops a healthy or mature brace of self-object relationships. For him or her—but overwhelmingly a him, which is why the male pronoun will be favored in many of the sentences that follow—self-object relationships are mostly "self-self" relationships that need to be intoxicating or that accommodate the narcissist's insatiable thirst for admiration.[11, p. 724] For this person, the last victory is indeed confirmation of his superiority and greatness, while his last defeat was utterly crushing (or a confabulatory "victory in disguise"). One type of very fragile narcissist is maniacally driven to keep on winning to convince himself of his self-worth, while a very advanced pathological narcissist, whose sense of self is absolute, might think: "Of course I won. Indeed, I shouldn't have even had to compete. They ought to have recognized my superiority straightaway and just given me the prize."

The Pathological Narcissist

Kohut and Kernberg both ascribe the unhealthy narcissist's pathology to parental empathic failures, but they differ on the ways these failures are appropriated by the child. For Kohut, narcissistic pathology begins when the parent consistently fails to respond appropriately to the child's need for mirroring and idealizing experiences.[12] It is interesting to note that the empathically inept parent might either overindulge the child or maintain an emotionally cold or distant relationship with the child. He or she may be either oppressively authoritarian or excessively permissive—a phenomenon that Watson and his colleagues empirically verified.[13] These phenomena can dispose the individual to developing an omnipotent self-image, which typically comes with unshakeable entitlement beliefs, or significant emotional insecurity which he or she compensates for by overachieving.

In either case, perhaps the hallmark characteristic of unhealthy narcissists is their insatiable need for respect, admiration, and adulation. To take an interesting historical example of such pathology, consider a passage from Harvey Sachs's biography of Arthur Rubinstein, one of the twentieth century's greatest concert pianists, wherein Sachs quotes Rubinstein's son John saying about his world famous father:

[T]here was a ferocity, a burning ferocity to my father's demand for adoring behavior; it was tough, possessive … I think that it had to do with how his mother and father had treated him, more than with how many people had heard his name or had written about him in the newspapers. In the only photo of my father's parents that I ever remember seeing, they look sort of bewildered. That's my one image of them. And perhaps he had some bewilderment in him, too—a feeling that 'no matter how much I surround myself with success, admirers, luxury, excitement, something is definitely missing.' For him, I believe, what was missing was a trust, a sense of being loved for himself, not for what he did or said; the kind of love that parents usually give you, and ironically, the kind that children usually give you … You couldn't love him enough for him to truly feel that trust. It was always subject to re-evaluation.[14, p. 310]

The photograph (taken in 1912) to which John Rubinstein referred is reproduced in the book and, rather than a look of bewilderment, the expressions on Izaak and Felicja Rubinstein faces seem to be emotional flatness, indifference, perhaps even smugness. They appear cold and distant, and it is worth noting that Rubinstein alternated between endearing and condescending comments about his parents throughout his life. In another passage, Sachs quotes Rubinstein's oldest child Eva offering a picture of the contradictory behaviors of her narcissistic father:

'He was not a normal child in his own house, among other children, among his own brothers and sisters; he immediately felt above them because he had a talent. The other children suddenly became inferior beings vis-à-vis their four-year-old brother, which is a very skewed sort of image of who's in charge,' … Thus, for the rest of his life, 'he had to be the center of attention, in control. This he could do: he was talented not only at music but also at storytelling, at getting everyone's attention … [but] Things had to go the way he saw them; when people didn't fit into his scheme of things, they became aliens or even enemies. If you disagreed about a book or a film, all of a sudden you were an idiot, having fifteen minutes before been the best, the most loved, the most intelligent: 'Ach, you're just like me, darling!' Which meant only, 'You agree with me,' even if you're just sitting there nodding because you don't dare say anything.[15, p. 305]

Virtually all theorists on narcissism posit that the infant as fetus experienced a state of uterine bliss to which the unhealthy narcissist pathologically longs to return.[16] The essence of "good-enough" parents consists in their ability to transition the child from the experience of having departed that wonderfully blissful and undifferentiated world (i.e., where the self was ALL that existed) to being able to manage the oppositionality of a world that is often utterly unaccommodating. What is central in that transition is for the parents to assist the child to integrate *both* positive and negative representations into his self-object representations.[17]

In contrast to Kohut's theory of narcissistic etiology, Otto Kernberg offered that the child did not so much experience a developmental lapse or injury, but rather reacted to the parental lack of empathy by accepting and identifying with it, resulting in his or her retaining as part of the psychic structure only those beliefs, feelings, and behaviors that the parent approved while repressing or discarding the rest.[18] Kernberg's model rests on his belief that the child-as-future-narcissist configures his or her behaviors explicitly to the parent's emotional manipulation so that the child's anxieties over his or her lovability can be calmed:

> [S]ometime between the ages of 3 and 5 years the narcissistic personality, instead of integrating positive and negative representations of self and object ... puts together all the positive representations and idealized representations of self and objects, which results in an extremely unrealistic and idealized concept of himself and a pathologic, grandiose self. He dissociates from himself, represses, or projects onto others all the negative aspects of himself and others. Fostering the development of a pathologic grandiose self are parents who are cold and rejecting, yet admiring. The narcissistic personality devaluates the real objects, having incorporated those aspects of the real objects that he wants for himself.[19, p. 724]

Children who sense their parents' emotional distance and are made insecure by it stand on a psychological precipice: If the child has no real or imagined resource by which he can prove his value and so secure the conditional love of the parent, he might succumb to the parental message that he is unlovable and will never amount to anything. These children often go on to purposefully avoid life situations that are in any way challenging because they are convinced of their failure and its accompanying emotional pain.[20] But children who, like Rubinstein, have confidence that they possess some personal asset that can be parlayed into approval or attention may well be on their way to a kind of "compensatory" narcissism—that is, a concentration of their self-formation around that skill, talent, or attribute so as to garner respect and attention that compensates them for the authentic, unconditional love they never experienced as children.[21] Later, these individuals can be suspicious of the affections of others since they do not know whether those affections occur conditionally or whether they are unconditional, that is, occur independently of whatever specialness the individual might display. Referring back to Rubinstein, we find his biographer Harvey Sachs saying:

> Throughout his life, however, Rubinstein worried that people loved him only for his talent—for what he was and not for who he was. 'WHEREVER did you get that neurosis that people don't love you for yourself????" exclaimed his old friend Mildred Knopf in 1978 after she had received a mournful telephone call from the ninety-one-year-old Rubinstein ... But .... he never quite believed such reassurances. His son John said, 'You couldn't love him enough.'[22, p. 11]

The Sadomasochistic Narcissist

An important facet of the narcissistic personality consists in how the narcissist cannot simply dismiss all those "objects" that cause him emotional pain because some of them might also be a source of his narcissistic supplies. A good example is the child-narcissist's parents, whom the child obviously cannot jettison from his life (although later he might come to hate them). The narcissist manages their presence by rationalizing their coldness and aloofness into something acceptable. In other words, he or she comes to confabulate the discomfort that is connected to his narcissistic supply as appropriate or deserved. Psychiatrist Arnold Cooper theorized that the narcissist's self-structure virtually has to admit a strongly masochistic dimension.[23] Thus, the immense capacity for hard work that is typical of many narcissists becomes transmogrified into a noble sacrifice, or something "crazy but cool," or as something they convince themselves is enjoyable. People who constantly derive and depend on intense narcissistic satisfaction from some object must be prepared for discouragement because no narcissistic supply is perfectly accommodating. Their psychological preparation, therefore, inevitably includes a conspicuous masochistic node that continues to affirm the validity of the narcissistic supply even though it also disappoints on occasion.

Also, as they cannot relate to themselves in an emotionally positive and healthy way, pathological narcissists are notable for finding it virtually impossible to evolve and sustain reciprocally loving relationships. Like Rubinstein, they understand experiential meaning only from their point of view. Moreover, many of them are unshakably convinced that personal achievement is the means of securing love and happiness, so that they proceed to sacrifice everything else—for example, their relationships with spouses, children, friends—to that end.[24] Consequently, if these narcissists do appear to have loving relationships with their significant others, it is largely because the latter have made immense sacrifices to enable them to realize their fantasies. Although married to his wife Nela for 50 years, Rubinstein was a remarkably tireless philanderer, apparently beginning his infidelities a few hours after his wedding ceremony in 1932. Yet, Nela, who made Rubinstein the center of her life, either ignored or simply refused to believe the rumors of his infidelities for 45 of the 50 years they were married. When they finally parted (but never divorced) a few years before his death so that he could continue an affair with a woman nearly 60 years his junior, he accused Nela of "never having loved him."[25, p. 371] In true narcissistic fashion, Rubinstein projected his own inability to sustain a deep and abiding love of others onto his wife. The narcissist is unable to understand how his own emotional dysfunction contributes to relational breakdowns.

Conclusion

Persons who are admirers of Rubinstein might be taken aback by the above musings on his narcissism, which serves to recall one of the prominent observations of Chapter 3:

Narcissism (like any personality disorder) is not a unitary phenomenon but admits numerous presentations. The reason, as Watson and his colleagues showed, is that narcissism is actually a bundle of traits, each of which has a certain magnitude. Moreover, some of these traits like emotional exploitativeness or unstable self-object relations are strongly associated with pathology, while others like assertiveness or leadership can correlate with a healthy self.[26]

The purely pathological narcissist is as rare as the individual who enjoys perfect emotional health. Most human beings fall somewhere between these poles and are a mix of negative and positive narcissistic traits. Thus, while this appendix depicts Rubinstein as a pointed example of an unhealthy narcissist, one might also counter that he was incredibly generous to his needy friends as well as to struggling musicians (even during his early years when he was often living hand to mouth); he was a tireless and immensely brave patriot for the Allies during World War II and later, an equally tireless supporter of the new state of Israel; he was an occasionally (although not always) magnificent father to his children; he derived immense enjoyment from warming the hearts of millions who heard him play; and he sustained lasting and devoted friendships throughout his very long life.

Crucial to the narcissistic personality's development in a healthy or unhealthy fashion is the quality of his or her self-esteem. And if Kohut, Kernberg, and Winnicott are right in emphasizing the significance of "good enough" parental empathy in the development of that esteem, then the eventual nature of an individual's narcissism is considerably dependent on forces external to him- or herself. Perhaps, too, certain children are in greater need of parental support and love than others so that their finding themselves in the midst of parentally deficient empathy spells a future self-developmental struggle. Indeed, here is where narcissism announces itself as not just an antidote but an *intoxicant* to which the individual might succumb and begin to develop those behavior patterns that disengage him or her from the felt experiences of others.

References

1. Ovid. *The Metamorphoses*. Trans. Horace Gregory, New York: The Viking Press, 1958, pp. 74–80.
2. Moore, Thomas. *Care of the Soul*. New York: HarperCollins, 1992.
3. Moore, 1992.
4. Masterson, James F. *The Search for the Real Self*. New York: The Free Press, 1988.
5. Akhtar, Salman. "Narcissistic personality disorder: Descriptive features and differential diagnosis." In *Narcissistic Personality Disorder. Psychiatric Clinics of North America*, ed. Otto Kernberg, 12(3):505–529, 1989.

6. Kernberg, Otto. "An ego psychology object relations theory of the structure and treatment of pathologic narcissism: An overview." In Kernberg, 1989. Kohut, Heinz. *Restoration of the Self.* New York: International Universities Press, 1977. For a more readable account of Kohut, see Goldberg, Arnold. "Self-psychology and the narcissistic personality disorders." In Kernberg, 1989, pp. 731–739.

7. Goldberg, 1989.

8. Winnicott, Donald W. *The Maturational Processes and the Facilitating Environment.* New York: International Universities Press, 1965.

9. Kernberg, Paulina. "Narcissistic personality disorder in childhood." In Kernberg, 1989, pp. 671–694.

10. Paulina Kernberg, 1989.

11. Otto Kernberg, 1989.

12. Goldberg, 1989.

13. Ramsey, Angela; Watson, Paul J.; Biderman, Michael D.; and Reeves, Amy l. "Self-reported narcissism and perceived parental permissiveness and authoritarianism." *The Journal of Genetic Psychology.* 157(2):227–238, 1996.

14. Sachs, Harvey. *Rubinstein: A Life.* New York: Grove Press, 1995.

15. Sachs, 1995.

16. Epstein, Mark. *thoughts without a thinker.* New York: Basic Books, 1995.

17. Paulina Kernberg, 1989.

18. Otto Kernberg, 1989.

19. Otto Kernberg, 1989.

20. Golomb, Elan. *Trapped in the Mirror.* New York: Quill, William Morrow, 1992.

21. Millon, Theodore. *Disorders of Personality: DSM-IV and Beyond.* New York: John Wiley & Sons, Inc., 1996, pp. 411–412.

22. Sachs, 1995.

23. Cooper, Arnold. "Narcissism and masochism: The narcissistic-masochistic character." In Otto Kernberg, 1989, pp. 541–552.

24. Millon, 1996.

25. Sachs, 1995.

26. Watson, Paul J.; Morris, Ronald J.; and Miller, Liv. "Narcissism and the self as continuum: Correlations with assertiveness and hypercompetitiveness." *Imagination, Cognition and Personality.* 17(3):249–259, 1997–98; Watson, Paul J.; Varnell, Sherri P.; and Morris, Ronald J. "Self-reported narcissism and perfectionism: An ego-psychological perspective and the continuum hypothesis." *Imagination, Cognition and Personality.* 19(1):59–69, 2000.

Index